MODELS IN CLINICAL NURSING:
THE WAY FORWARD

To Anne Kathryn, my daughter, with all my love

MODELS IN CLINICAL NURSING: THE WAY FORWARD

MIKE WALSH

BA(Hons), RGN, PGCE, DipN(Lond)
Senior Lecturer in Nursing
St Martin's College, Lancaster UK

with contributions by:

June Andrews MA, RMN, RGN, RCN Advisor on
AIDS, Royal College of Nursing, London UK

Cathy Ashmore RGN, DN, PWT, Cert.Ed FE, Senior Lecturer in Community Nursing,
Bristol Polytechnic, Bristol UK

Miriam Rosewell BSc, MSc, RGN, Lecturer of Nursing, King's College, University of London, London UK

Baillière Tindall
London   Philadelphia   Toronto   Sydney   Tokyo

Baillière Tindall   24–28 Oval Road
W.B. Saunders   London NW1 7DX

The Curtis Center
Independence Square West
Philadelphia, PA 19106–3399, USA

55 Horner Avenue
Toronto, Ontario, M8Z 4X6, Canada

Harcourt Brace Jovanovich Group (Australia) Pty Ltd
30–52 Smidmore Street
Marrickville
NSW 2204, Australia

Harcourt Brace Jovanovich Japan Inc
Ichibancho Central Building, 22–1 Ichibancho
Chiyoda-ku, Tokyo 102, Japan

Typeset by Columns Design and Production Services Ltd, Reading, England
Printed in Great Britain by Thomson Litho Ltd, East Kilbride, Scotland

British Library Cataloguing in Publication Data is available

ISBN 0–7020–1560–1

CONTENTS

Acknowledgements

To June Andrews for helping with the chapter on mental health; the library staff of the Avon College of Nursing and Midwifery, Bristol Centre for their help and forebearance while I was researching the book, and finally to Helen Chalmers and Peter Aggleton who first taught me about nursing models and made me realize their potential value while I was studying for the London Diploma in Nursing at Bath a long time ago.

INTRODUCTION

In writing this book the aim has been to relate theoretical models of nursing to the real world of clinical practice. This is not an erudite and abstruse text, but rather an attempt to tackle the issues of planning and delivering high-quality care at a time when nursing is facing a major threat to its autonomy coupled with grave difficulties of staffing and resourcing. It will be argued that while there are problems and difficulties in working with models, there are also potentially great benefits which nursing cannot afford to ignore for the sake of patients as well as nurses.

The focus of the book is on a series of mainstream models — those of Orem, Roy, Roper, King — and the use of the FANCAP assessment tool. High standards of nursing care require the use of individualized care planning, the so-called nursing process, and this is discussed in conjunction with the various models. In addition to looking at general adult hospital care the book has incorporated a view from the community of models and care planning. The major speciality of oncology has also been studied, firstly to show that there is a place for models in specialized nursing and also because cancer patients will be encountered by nurses in a wide range of settings. Finally, the role of models in the very different world of mental illness has been addressed and it has been shown how flexibility allows the integration of the FANCAP scheme with King's model of nursing in this area.

The care plans offered in this book are not presented as the definitive way of caring for a patient who has had a certain type of surgery or who who is recovering from some medical crisis such as a myocardial infarction. Rather they are offered as ways of using a nursing model to plan care that is patient centred in a rational way. They are offered as examples of how to document model-based care that will hopefully help the reader towards achieving good quality care plans and most importantly, better quality care in practice.

It is time to draw the boundaries of nursing and say how we operate within those boundaries. Nursing models are the stuff of nursing and as such are key components in this process, although as the text argues, they need development and refinement as a result of practice. Nursing cannot exist as a practice without a theoretical base to grow from just as a forest cannot exist without soil and water. A flexible and dynamic approach is needed towards the development of a whole series of models. There is no place for dogma and one model only!

It is time we broke free of the 'Doubting Thomas' approach, the cynics and head shakers, the 'Little Englanders' who oppose models of nursing simply because they originate in the United States. It is a time to be brave and have a go at developing the profession of nursing into the next century instead of sitting timidly in the shadow of general management and medical domination. As a 'Child of the 60s' the author is often reminded of Bob Dylan's classic song 'The Times they are a-Changin', I have that feeling about nursing now. These are very fundamental and deep changes that go to the very roots of what nursing is and who controls it. It is a time for nursing theory if we are to define what nursing practice is and hence be able to justify our direct patient care.

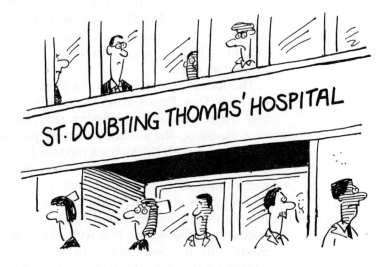

1 CHOOSING A MODEL OF NURSING

Do models really matter?

Before asking the reader to invest time and effort in the study of how to apply models of nursing to patient care, we must first of all establish that they actually are important and worthwhile. After all, we have been nursing in the UK since the days of Nightingale without the nursing models of people such as Roy, Orem and Roper, so why do we need them now?

Authors such as Hardy (1986) clearly feel that nursing can do without models because they lead to incomprehensible jargon and 'tramlines' thinking where nurses see only what a model tells them to see, leading to a lack of questioning and a failure to recognize individuals for their true worth. Hardy further argues that a model is subjective: it is only one person's view of the world and it is therefore wrong to design a nursing care plan around such a single view.

Hardy's views, however, are flawed. Nursing has had jargon ever since there has been nursing; models are not to blame for that, although the difficult language that some authors use invites criticism. Listen carefully to the language used at the next shift handover to see how nurses use jargon. It is said that the excessive use of American expressions makes some models incomprehensible, yet that does not detract from the popularity enjoyed by American TV programmes and films amongst nurses and the rest of the population!

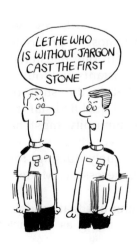

LET HE WHO IS WITHOUT JARGON CAST THE FIRST STONE

The issue of rigid thinking leading to ritualistic practice is a serious problem facing nursing today, and as Walsh and Ford (1989) have shown, this has many causes, but nursing models do not figure in their list. Rather the challenges and questions thrown down by the development of nursing models should open nurses' minds and lead to research and whole new ways of thinking about and practising nursing.

A model may represent the author's own view of nursing, but gravity represented Newton's way of thinking about the world, the heart as a pump circulating blood around the body was Harvey's way of thinking and of course Relativity was Einstein's personal view of the universe. There is nothing wrong therefore in a framework of

3

ideas coming from one individual head, providing those ideas are disseminated widely and worked upon by others to see how well they explain the real world.

The examples quoted here are of course from the physical sciences; nursing, however, deals with a more intangible field of endeavour — human behaviour. Consider others who have pronounced upon human behaviour, from the Ancient Greeks such as Plato through to the philosophers and revolutionaries of modern history. Where would the United States be if the views of Washington and the Founding Fathers had been ignored because they were subjective? The ideas of Churchill and Roosevelt helped defeat Nazi tyranny, itself the product of one man's subjective views. The individual can therefore have profound effects upon human behaviour on a global scale, but that individual also has to be in the right place at the right time; there has to be a major groundswell of change occurring within a society before an individual's views can take a hold. History is much much more than famous names and events.

Perhaps that is how it is in nursing today; there is a groundswell of change after a century of the medical model being in the ascendancy. Circumstances are combining today to bring forward radically different views of nursing, and the development of nursing models is one way in which these new ideas are being articulated. To go back to Hardy's criticism that models are subjective, yes they are in their present stage of development, but they are none the worse for that!

Models really do matter because they are the stuff of nursing. If we are to argue that nursing is a profession in its own right, then we need to be able to work out the boundaries of nursing so that we can recognize our legitimate field of practice. If nurses wish to be able to deliver the quality of care that they feel patients deserve, they must first of all know what that care is and how it should be delivered in order that they can fight for the necessary resources to carry out that care. The struggle for resources has become an increasingly dominant feature of the UK health scene in recent years and nursing care is the biggest consumer of those scarce resources.

Arguments about skill mix and staffing levels on wards revolve around what needs to be done and who is the most appropriate person to carry out that care. Can wards be run with one registered nurse and the rest of the staff acting as care assistants without a professional qualification? If not, why not? What is the stuff of nursing that says this cannot be, that it needs several qualified staff to care for these patients or that patients in the community must be visited by registered nurses? In attempting to answer these sort of questions we are trying to define that which is uniquely nursing, for which a professional education and qualification is necessary. Models of nursing are trying to do the same thing.

Field (1987) has argued along these lines, pointing out that models and theories indicate the area of practice that is nursing as distinct from that of other allied health professionals. Nursing of course draws on these allied areas such as medicine or the behavioural sciences, but the nurse needs to take such knowledge and interpret it in nursing terms for it to be of benefit to the patient. Thus, Field rightly cautions that nursing models alone do not provide a sufficient knowledge base for nursing care, rather they set the framework for knowledge from a range of disciplines to be synthesized into effective nursing care. Nursing models are thus essential as they map out the boundaries of nursing and facilitate the bringing together of knowledge from a wide range of other disciplines to supplement the core nursing knowledge required for quality nursing care.

It is only possible to defend something when its boundaries are known, and today we need to defend nursing from the threats of de-skilling and take-over by a whole range of specialist technicians. Models define those boundaries and help us organize our delivery of care to suit the patients' needs.

Luker (1988) in asking whether models will work or not raised the question that they may be red herrings. Nurses might say they have implemented a model, leading to the belief that change has occurred and gaining academic kudos in the process. This could be an illusion, though and in reality very little has altered apart from using different bits of paper and introducing some new jargon. The obvious analogy with the implementation of the nursing process will be discussed later. For now we should observe that introducing a model requires a fundamental re-examination of the way we think and carry out nursing care. Anything less is merely academic window dressing and cannot be given credit as really tackling the challenges presented by nursing models.

Do models matter? If having a theory influences practice, then yes they matter. Torres (1986) pointed out that just as models of teaching or psychology influence the practice of these disciplines, so too it is with nursing, while Botha (1989) considers that the influence of theories of nursing upon practice is so self-evident that it no longer needs argument. This sweeping statement cannot be left unchallenged and Kristjanson *et al.* (1987) indeed take issue with this view, arguing that the literature contains no evidence that different conceptual frameworks produce differences in practice. Recent work by Faucett (Faucett *et al.*, 1990) does, however, suggest that implementing a model of nursing, in this case Orem's Self Care model, does produce changes in practice and for the better. A fuller consideration of Faucett's work will be found later (p. 31). For now the case will be argued that, as practice cannot be divorced from theory in any discipline, models of nursing do matter!

What are models of nursing?

Certain words in this debate tend to be tossed around interchangeably, such as models, theories and conceptual frameworks. They do have different meanings which should be investigated at this stage. A concept is an idea, so a conceptual framework is a pattern of ideas. Such a widely accepted pattern of ideas is known sometimes as a paradigm, for example the framework of ideas that seeks to explain how we learn might be called a paradigm.

In defining models it is best to think of them as simplified ways of representing reality, as ways to facilitate understanding. They can be numerical models suitable for computers that seek to show how a complex system such as the atmosphere works or othey can be physical models such as the anatomy models we are all familiar with from our basic training. Models can also be built with ideas, and in dealing with nursing models we are looking at sets of ideas that represent and try and give an understanding of what nursing consists of.

Theories can also be constructed from ideas but they are much tighter structures than models for they try to explain relationships between things in a deterministic way, i.e. if this happens then this will follow; there are therefore law-like elements of generalization and prediction involved in theories. Given this structure, it is possible to test theories with experimental observation. A hypothesis can be derived from the theory and this hypothesis examined experimentally; if the hypothesis fails then the theory is open to serious doubt, but if it is successfully confirmed, then this supports the theory although it is not necessarily proof. Scientists are very wary of the word proof; such are the limitations of experimental method it is not usually possible to be so absolute as to say X proves Y. Proof in the strict sense occurs only in the abstract world of mathematics. This approach is known as the hypothetico-deductive method. For example, Newton's theory of gravitation led to the hypothesis that two objects of equal weight, no matter what they are composed of, will in a vacuum fall at the same rate. This has been tested and confirmed both in laboratories and by astronauts on the moon.

Which is the correct terminology to apply in nursing? Given the complexity of human behaviour it is unlikely that nursing will ever be able to produce theories with all the characteristics discussed above and it is better to talk of models or conceptual frameworks. To talk of theories of nursing implies that there are hypotheses about nursing that can be derived and experimentally tested from such work, a questionable assertion to say the least. For a view of nursing to rejoice in the title of theory it needs to be generalizable to many practice fields and be capable of prediction, which as Kristjanson *et al.* (1987) point out is not the case at present, leading these authors to argue against the view that nursing models are true theories. They also wisely argue against the implementation of any single nursing model as the definitive method of carrying out nursing for this reason. We will return to this point later (p. 9) when model choice is discussed.

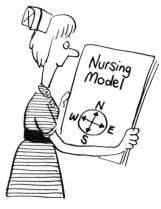

A model of nursing offers us a way of thinking about nursing. It is rather like a map and compass in that it maps out the terrain of nursing; it gives the nursing–patient interaction structure and allows us to find our way around this complex topography. Perhaps today we are at the stage of having carried out the first rough survey of the ground; we have only a sketch map showing a major river here and a mountain there, but we are awaiting the Ordnance Survey to come along and give us a reliable, detailed map that will allow us to confidently trust any chosen nursing model. It is up to nurses to be their own surveyors, however, and not allow others to map out our territory for us: we must be our own Ordnance Survey.

The reliable charting of the model will only come from nurses working with the model, trying it out, questioning it and suggesting adaptations and improvements. Models are not set in tablets of stone, but rather are loose frameworks of ideas whose aim is to facilitate care, not to get in the way. Wright (1986) has written about the way a model of nursing evolved on his care of the elderly unit from the ideas of Virginia Henderson coupled with the development of existing practice by the unit staff. This is an excellent example of the usage of nursing models.

This approach involves starting out with a framework of ideas and putting them into practice, and observing how they perform before adapting them to try to achieve better results. This contrasts with the hypothetico-deductive method described above and is known as inductive reasoning, whereby generalizations and knowledge are generated from observation (Pollit and Hungler, 1985). Thus, Orem's Self Care model (1985) leads us to expect that patients with diabetes would wish to learn how to manage their diabetes for themselves; however, observing real patients shows this is sometimes not the case, therefore we must think why not? What causes these exceptions? How can we adapt this model of nursing to accommodate this observation and help patients who are poorly controlling their diabetes to manage their health more effectively? This is inductive reasoning working within a nursing model to adapt and refine that model.

Is it possible to generate a model of nursing from pure observation with no preconceived ideas? The answer is no, because such an inductive system needs an original framework of ideas and concepts, for as Hammersley and Atkinson (1983) points out, it is impossible to discover the nature of the social world without some method to guide our practice. Nursing models, with their views about the nature of people, how nurses and patients interact, the environment surrounding this interaction and the nature of health and illness serve to provide this framework.

Field (1987) has developed this idea and argues that as long as any model includes these four key elements plus a method of systematic problem solving (the nursing process) then it can rightly be considered a nursing model. What will differ, however, is the way in which the data base is organized, i.e. how the assessment differs, leading to different nursing diagnoses and hence differing approaches to care. Field therefore argues that differing nursing models will lead to differences in care and illustrates her case with reference to a comparison of Orem's, Neuman's and Roy's models.

Field sees nurse theorists as thinkers who on the basis of years of practical experience have tried to break nursing down into the constituent parts that go to make up the whole and in this way give nursing a theoretical framework. There is a danger here and, as Botha (1989) points out, the theorist may come to deal only in the abstract, leading to the risk of reductionism. Thus, the theorist loses touch with reality as the complexities of every day life become broken down into convenient, easy to handle packages and the human factor becomes lost. Rourke (1990) is very critical of the Roper model from this point of view because it leads to ritualistic nursing as the patient is dehumanized into a series of biological systems, some of which are seen as failing. Roper's model is therefore constructed in such a way that it only focuses on negative physical attributes, leading to patient labelling and ignoring the psychological and social aspects of the person.

Nursing models, therefore, are not watertight theories, but rather sets of ideas about the way patients and nurses interact. The dangers of reductionism and losing touch with reality are such that model development must take place with at least one foot in the real world of practical nursing care. Model development and nursing practice should therefore be closely related by continual feedback, and both should never lose sight of the person as a holistic integrated being.

Choosing a model It is necessary to look first at the different types of model that are available before considering how to choose between them.

In the preceding section we saw that it is unlikely that there will ever be one general nursing model that will be satisfactory for all situations. Human behaviour is too complex for that and if theorists try to develop increasingly abstract and general models in an attempt to explain everything, they will end up explaining nothing (Miller 1985 in Wright, 1986). This therefore means that inevitably there will be many different types of model from which the nurse has to choose.

This is a healthy state of affairs for any discipline, as competing approaches to problems stimulate debate, enquiry and research, whereas a single solution leads to minds being closed against alternatives and the triumph of the procedure manual over individualized, creative nursing care. Botha (1989) has argued passionately for the development of a variety of models as in her view the proliferation of theories opens up any discipline and equips its practitioner to deal with a wide range of situations. As Kristjanson *et al.* (1987) point out, the adoption of a single universal model of nursing stultifies critical appraisal of that model and leads to a single approach to nursing being used that is lacking in evidence to support its validity.

Hardy (1986) has described the parlous state of affairs that can arise when a single model of nursing is adopted to the exclusion of all others, leading to a situation where lip service only is paid to the model, which nobody actually believes in. She reminds us of the work of Peters and Waterman (1982), who wrote a classic account of what makes for a successful business. They found it was the avoidance of rigid management models and instead a bias for action out of which creativity could flow, emphasis on the importance of people and 'staying close to the customer' to provide service of the highest quality.

In terms of using models of nursing, therefore, we must beware the zealots who would have one model only to the exclusion of all others. Sadly UK nursing seems to show signs of this approach with the blanket implementation of the much criticized Roper model. Nursing must avoid reducing models to ritualistic exercises in bureaucracy; rather, clinicians must have the freedom to develop and evolve models in the light of practical experience; only in this way can the notions of creativity and staying close to the customer espoused by Peters and Waterman work to the full benefit of all concerned.

It must also be said that, in view of the immature state of many nursing models, the more they are used and compared with each other, the better will be the likely outcome as inductive reasoning is used to develop and refine each model in turn. Cross-fertilization can also occur as nurses borrow concepts and ideas from one model and apply them to another. Field (1987) has defended models from the charge of incompleteness in these very terms, arguing that attempts to negate the role they can play in nursing is an unfortunate and uninformed attitude when what is needed is constructive usage.

It can, however, be a daunting prospect for the nurse to be confronted by a dozen or more different models of nursing and to have to decide which ones are suitable for her or his own clinical area. It might help nurses, therefore, to stop and think in broad terms about what type of model would be most applicable to their nursing situation before getting into the detail of individual models. At this broad strategic level the writings of Aggleton and Chalmers (1987) are most useful as they show that models can be grouped under three broad headings, developmental, systems and interactionist.

A developmental model will focus on how a person is developing and how nursing is needed when normal development is threatened or actually impaired. Development refers to more than the obvious physical aspects of human behaviour and also includes psychological

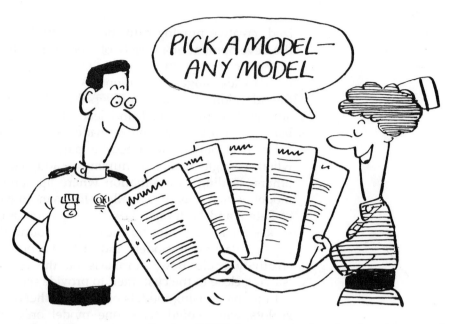

and social processes. Peplau (1952) is an example of a developmental approach, but strong developmental strands can be found in other models such as that of Orem (1985).

The systems approach is concerned not only with physiological systems but also with psychological and social systems, and how they all interact. Notions of maintaining balance between systems run through such models as the body strives for homeostasis; consequently, nursing is seen in these terms, i.e. helping the person achieve equilibrium or a balance of functioning in their everyday life. Roy (1984) and King (1981) are examples of systems models, although the latter has a strong interactionist component.

An interactionist view of nursing centres around how humans communicate with each other and the meanings that are attached to such communication. Striving to see the other person's point of view and understand the role they are playing are essential ingredients of such models as patients are seen to have health problems deriving from self-perception and the roles they are adopting in living their life. Riehl (1980) and Orlando (1961) have offered models of nursing based upon these interactionist principles.

Aggleton and Chalmers emphasize that these three broad categories of models are not mutually exclusive. A nursing model can lie largely in one area, but still borrow ideas from the others. Thus, Orem sees the need for self-care as the core of her model and requires the nurse to assess the patient's self-care ability in a physiological systems manner, but her model also requires an assessment of the patient's developmental status, as this clearly affects self-care ability. The model may also be enhanced by asking the nurse to consider how the patients see their self-care requirements — their point of view may be very different from the nurse's. For example, while the nurse may consider smoking as harmful to health and therefore a self-care failure, the patient may see this as helpful to self-care as it is perceived to reduce stress.

If an integrated and holistic approach to nursing is to be developed, it seems logical not to rely exclusively on just one of the types of model identified by Aggleton and Chalmers. We have already seen how concentration on systems leads to a reductionist and dehumanizing approach in the case of Roper, yet if only an interactionist approach were used, how might this be applied to a patient capable of little or no interaction with the nurse, e.g. an unconscious patient? In developing and applying models of nursing it is therefore essential that we recognize the need for the three dimensions of systems homeostasis, developmental status and nurse–patient interaction to be incorporated into any working model. The nurse may start out with a model that is, for example, predominantly systems oriented, but should aim to incorporate into its application a developmental and interactionist perspective. For example, in assessing the patient after choosing a systems model, the nurse may choose to consider for each topic the effect of the patient's age and position on the continuum of life and also how the patient sees and interprets events. In this way a more rounded picture of the patient emerges.

In practice, however, the nurse can only choose from what is on the menu and that means choosing an established model that will have a strong bias towards systems and homeostasis, developmental status or interactionism. The nurse therefore needs to consider how much his or her nursing practice is about restoring equilibrium and balance to permit everyday living, or whether the prime objective is to foster development and growth or to help a person understand how their perceptions of life and the roles they choose to act may be contributing to their health problems. These broad strategic aims and the sort of patients that are going to be cared for need to be thought through before homing in on any one group of models. The nurse therefore needs to work out a philosophy of care and the models must be matched to the philosophy, not the other way round. Nursing care cannot be forced into models like square pegs in round holes.

Arriving at a philosophy of care

The phrase 'philosophy of care' has a rather academic ring to it, but all it really means is what the basic beliefs are that underpin our approach to nursing. Such beliefs depend to some extent on the way we see life in general and also the way we see the delivery of health care. A philosophy of care might cover a ward, a unit or a community team and should be derived from the views of all the staff who work in that area and, wherever possible, the patients as well.

Wright (1986) has given a good account of how his unit developed

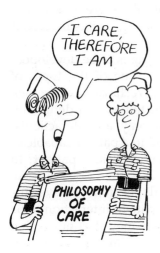

their philosophy out of a series of meetings that involved all the staff on the unit as well as the views of the patients. For example, part of the philosophy states that each patient is seen as an individual entitled to the highest-quality skilled nursing care on an equal footing with any other person regardless of race, colour or creed and also entitled to freedom of choice in determining that care.

In determining a philosophy, general principles such as this need to be combined with the more specific needs of patients. Thus, patients in a hospice for the terminally ill will have some different needs from patients in a unit for the mentally ill, while acute hospital patients will have some different needs from community patients. The nurse can think of many different care settings and see that while there may be a common core to a philosophy involving the sort of values we cherish in a Western democracy such as those outlined by Wright above, there will also be some more specific elements dependent upon the type of care setting.

It is essential to enter a word of warning here, however. Supposing the patient does not subscribe to the nursing philosophy? An obvious example might be the way women are perceived in some cultures that are very different from the culture of northern Europe. Even within that latter culture there are many variations in how men, and women, see the woman's role.

To some extent this problem can be reduced by ensuring that patients are fully involved in drawing up a philosophy in the first place and by trying to make that philosophy as broad as possible to accommodate different points of view. However, it is still likely that there may be a problem of the nursing view being different from that of some patients. The nursing team need to debate the notion that, at the end of the day, the patient is always right, even if the nurse disagrees with the patient. This philosophical problem underlines the need for the nursing team to look at the interactionist approach to nursing and grapple with the patient's point of view.

It must be emphasized that the philosophy should be derived from the efforts of all members of the care team. There is nothing more destructive than having different members of a team pulling in different directions or playing a game by different rules from everybody else. All team members must feel able to subscribe to a philosophy of care if it is to succeed, which means they must all be fully and equally involved in working out that philosophy. If each person feels that there is a little piece of his or herself in the philosophy, the team will come to own the philosophy; it will be seen as 'ours', which in turn helps to develop commitment and participation.

The philosophy should therefore reflect the patients' and care team's general views about human rights and health, and also ideas specific to the needs of the patients to be cared for, having been derived from the efforts of all staff and patients.

Matching the model to the philosophy

Once a clear idea has emerged of the nursing philosophy, the next step is to look at the types of models that are available before moving on to look at specific, individual models. As we have seen, models can focus on developmental aspects, on maintaining a balance between systems to ensure satisfactory human functioning or on interactionism, seeing things from patient's point of view.

The three approaches discussed above may all appear equally attractive at first sight, but after careful consideration and discussion with colleagues and patients it should be possible to see one approach a little ahead of the others as being most appropriate. Having decided which of these three stratagems seems best, the nurse should not shut his or her mind to what the alternatives have to offer, but consider how much of these other approaches to nursing might also be taken on board. After all, a cake baked from flour, fat and water would be very dull and unsatisfactory, but add smaller proportions of some other very different ingredients such as chocolate and cream and the result is very different.

The next step is to try to pick a single model out from one of these three broad areas, always remembering what aspects associated with other types of models would be helpful also. This is essential as, when trying to make our chosen model work, we can adapt and change it accordingly. For example, we may have chosen a systems model such as Roy's, but the nursing team may feel it is very important to know the patient's point of view at all times, reflecting the interactionist approach. Arguments have been deployed in favour of a multi-model approach to nursing (p. 9), so the reader might detect a contradiction at this stage. The answer is that we should learn to walk before we run, as for most nurses the notion of models is a new concept, and therefore it is important not to be over-ambitious to start with. The aim should be to get one model of nursing working in a unit, then this can be adapted, changed and developed by the inductive process discussed earlier.

Parallel developments could see other models being introduced in other areas and perhaps, after a year or more the differing models would have been 'run in' sufficiently (like a new car) to allow nurses to ask two very important questions. Firstly, has model X improved care in my unit? Secondly, what other models could be introduced from other areas into my clinical patch? Answers to these two questions depend amongst other things upon evaluation of the quality of care given.

The aim would be over a 2–3-year period to have several different models working in one care setting. Differing units may have each pioneered a different model on their own wards, but after this initial development period it is to be hoped that models would spread across wards and eventually any one ward may be able to offer several different approaches to care, selecting the one most appropriate to each individual patient.

At this stage it has to be acknowledged that it appears that a great deal of responsibility for developing and implementing nursing models is being placed upon clinical staff. Is this fair or realistic given all the other pressures staff face just to keep the service going? The disastrous implementation of the nursing process serves as a red light which should tell us to stop here and consider carefully exactly how staff on a busy ward or community patch can realistically be expected to implement a nursing model.

Implementing a model

Many writers have commented upon the disastrous way that the nursing process was foisted upon nursing in the UK (Walsh and Ford, 1989) with top-down implementation by a management that did not understand the basic concepts of care planning. Such a poorly managed change exercise guaranteed failure as the nursing process was greeted with hostility and scepticism. Laughlin (1988) and Lister (1987) are only two of many to draw an analogy with models, for if their attempted implementation follows the same pattern, the result will be equally disastrous. They argue that change should not occur for change's sake and that the imposition of models would be a great mistake. How right they are, for models will only find their way into nursing practice if nurses can see advantages in their introduction and can feel fully involved in their development.

This requires a bottom-up approach to models and not top-down implementation from either managers or academics. The original impetus towards introducing a model might come from a member of the ward team who develops an interest in the topic through a post-basic course or by attending a study day or reading a journal article or book. A new member of staff may join the ward who has studied models as part of an undergraduate training programme or the subject might be raised at a unit meeting. A key person in a ward or unit introducing a model of nursing is the charge nurse or sister, the acknowledged leader of the clinical team, and it is from within that team that the drive to change must be developed.

The Project 2000 reform of education seems set to introduce models of nursing into the basic nurse curriculum, but do tutors have sufficient grasp of the ideas and concepts involved to be able to teach about different models? This is a worrying gap in nurse education at present and one which it is hoped tutors and colleges will make strenuous efforts to close.

A recurring criticism of nurse education involves the fact that what students are taught in school often bears little resemblance to the reality of clinical areas. Teaching of models in colleges of nursing when they are not encountered in practice seems set to perpetuate this chronic problem. Morales-Mann and Logan (1990) offer interesting insights into the difficulties of designing a nurse education programme around models of nursing. They describe how the School of Nursing at the University of Ottawa decided to base its nursing curriculum upon a pluralistic approach to models, starting with the Roy model for the first year of the course. Before utilizing Roy's model, however, it was rigorously tested against the criteria of compatibility with the needs of the students, completeness as a model, praticality and feasibility. Only when it had met these criteria was the model chosen for use.

The use of Roy in this way required a fundamental rethink of the first-year curriculum, the teaching of supporting subjects to be congruent with Roy's model, the development of new teaching aids and a great deal of work to familiarize ward staff with the concepts involved. It was opposition from the ward staff that represented the greatest obstacle to change and presented the greatest difficulty to teaching the students Roy's model. Personal experience in teaching nursing undergraduates to use the Roy model (and other models) while working in clinical areas that adhere to traditional medical model nursing or that pay lip service to the Roper approach supports the views of Morales-Mann and Logan. Before colleges of nursing implement a multi-model curriculum, a great deal of care and attention must be paid to thinking through which models are most appropriate to what areas of the course; recognition must be paid to the effects on how other areas of the course are taught as well as the effects on nursing teaching; and finally the problem must be addressed of how the students will cope with gaining experience on wards that are not using the models being taught in college.

This leads to the proposal that models need to be introduced in clinical practice with a bottom-up approach, and until they are working in at least a substantial part of the clinical field their value in basic nurse education will be limited to that of an academic exercise. However, it is to be hoped that, as more nurses qualify with a knowledge of nursing models, implementation into clinical areas will accelerate so that eventually students will indeed be able to practise nursing in the way they have been taught in college.

One further impetus to model development might therefore be from within the college of nursing, as teaching models will only be good educational practice if they are being used in clinical areas. It would be wrong to say that unless a ward is using a model students will not be sent there for clinical experience and that therefore the ward must adopt a model immediately. Such a quick fix solution will lead to lip service only being paid to any model, like the nursing process, and the rationale for model choice will be expediency. The model chosen will represent the lowest common denominator that requires least understanding. The easiest model to understand is not always the best, after all it is much easier to understand that the earth is flat and that the sun goes around the earth, but both these models of the solar system are very wrong.

Nurse educators are therefore important change agents and along with clinical staff make up the two most likely sources for the impetus to introduce a model. However, to be effective they must be much more closely involved with the clinical field and work together with clinical staff in model development. We will return to this point later.

Introducing a model to a clinical area is not a task to be undertaken lightly, as it involves fundamental changes in the way staff think and work. Luker (1988) has suggested that each nurse carries around their own informal model of nursing which guides their practice. It is probable that a formal model will be significantly different, although these differences can be minimized by full consultation and involvement with staff to ensure that the model chosen reflects their views of nursing as far as possible.

It is interesting to compare Luker's notion of each nurse carrying around their own personal model of nursing with the ideas of Benner (1984), who discusses the way nurses evolve from novices through the stages of advanced beginner, competency, proficiency and expertise. The key to this development is the nurse's evolution from adherence to rigid patterns of formal rules in the novice stage through more flexible and analytical thinking patterns to a final stage of problem solving that appears to an outsider as intuitive, so effectively have thought patterns become internalized. The expert nurse seems to automatically know the answer!

Luker's experienced nurses with their own personal model contained in their head may be equated with Benner's expert nurse. The problem arises in that very often an expert nurse cannot explain the process of their nursing, which has become based on this internalized personal model which, as Field (1987) points out, limits the development of the practice base of the profession. Two salient features emerge from these considerations. Firstly, the development of expertise depends upon patterning of knowledge and experience; therefore to promote expertise we need to promote that patterning process. Models of nursing help to provide a framework and pattern for nursing and therefore should be encouraged since they can assist a nurse's professional development. The second point addresses Luker's personal models: if every nurse has a different model of nursing, which as Benner argues will be largely implicit and appear intuitive, how can we share and develop nursing expertise? The need is for a common language or at least a common framework to allow clinical experts to share their knowledge with others rather than pursue their implicit, apparently intuitive, internal model of nursing.

Benner's concept of the novice nurse sticking closely to rigid rules is of relevance to educationalists and clinical staff who might be involved in a models-based, pre-registration educational programme. The author's personal experience in teaching on just such a course confirms Benner's views of how novices and beginners function, particularly with reference to models of nursing. Students seem to want a comprehensive assessment scheme that has a neat pigeonhole for every aspect of the patient, leading to difficulties in working with

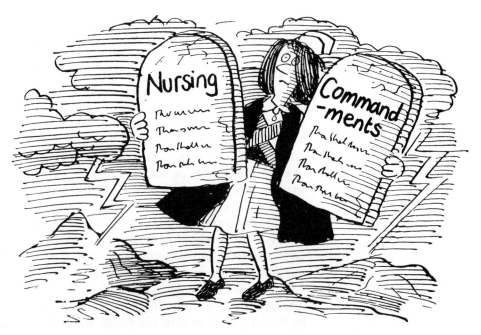

models such as Roy or Orem and particularly the FANCAP scheme (see p. 75), where the nurse is required to be flexible and interpret patient behaviour so as to assign it a place in the assessment scheme. A rigid, simplistic approach simply will not work and it must be recognized that the nurse has to move on along the scale of proficiency before being able to synthesize and analyse information in such a way as to make maximum use of any model. Nursing education must be aware of this, with the notion of the spiral curriculum being a valid tool in this context, extending education beyond registration level.

Consider the example of pain; although there is no heading specifically entitled 'pain' under Roy, Orem or Roper, it still may be assessed. However, students frequently criticize these models because there is no such explicit heading in the assessment schedule, finding it difficult to see that the notion of body regulation and adaptation found in Roy's model directs the nurse to think of the nervous system, which in turn should lead to consideration of sensation and pain. Orem's health deviancy self-care category should also make the nurse enquire about pain, a very common symptom of 'health deviancy' to use Orem's slightly clumsy phrase. Pain can be seen as a dimension of Roper's activities of living, e.g. it may be associated with mobilizing or breathing, and as such may be introduced wherever appropriate in the assessment. An assessment format that was as explicit as many junior students request would be totally unwieldy and fragment the patient beyond recognition in a battery of headings and subheadings.

It would therefore benefit students to introduce them early in their education to models that do have a more explicit assessment tool, such as Roper or Henderson, leaving other models until later. As students gain knowledge and experience they will be better able to interpret and use the more implicit assessment tools of other models which require higher-level functioning.

In developing models as a common language of nursing, creativity and individualism are to be encouraged and this is no argument for conformity in approaches to nursing. However, if nursing models were more used and well known, they could offer a common framework of ideas within which expert nurses could make more explicit the secrets of their success. A process of reflection, of looking at what the nurse does and placing successful care in a theoretical framework, could be of immense benefit to nursing. The experienced stoma care nurse may be able to benefit others by using Roy's model to try to understand how she successfully helps the patient to adapt to the stoma, while the experienced psychiatric nurse may be able to explain her success in helping a patient return to the home environment by analysing care using the concepts of King. It is about interpreting the individual nurse's implicit model in terms of an explicit model that is in the public domain and has common meanings to most nurses.

Use of a model will also bring other changes in its wake, for, as we shall see in the next chapter, full implementation of individualized care planning (i.e. the nursing process) will be necessary along with primary nursing.

Introducing a model is therefore a major exercise in changing attitudes and beliefs, as well as practice. Attitudes are very difficult to change, as people regard them as part of themselves, their own bit of property, consequently they tend to hang on to them. Nursing is very bad at letting people fail, yet to change and try out new ideas staff must feel able to fail, for mistakes are an inevitable part of the change process.

The social sciences offer us one method of changing attitudes that has been shown to work. It rejoices in the grand title of cognitive dissonance theory and it is really saying that people always tend to try to reconcile what they believe with what they know. Therefore, to change beliefs, the need is to change experience, for that determines what we know. The racial integration of American society in the 1960s was partly accomplished on the basis of this theory, which predicted that if white people came to experience and therefore know black people, they would be faced by the problem of reconciling their prejudiced old beliefs with a new reality that would often be very different. The way this might happen is by changing their beliefs to fit their new knowledge. To some extent this is indeed what happened and, while there is still a great deal of racial tension in the United States today, the situation is a lot better than it was 30 years ago.

This principle applied to nursing suggests that after a period of intensive debate and work involving all the staff, there has to come a time when a unit moves forward and implements its chosen model. Staff still displaying negative attitudes can experience working with the new system and, along with help and support, they will have to face reconciling a great deal of positive experience with their negative beliefs, which it is hoped will lead to a shift in belief.

The introduction of change in nursing has been shown by Hunt (1987) to require a great deal of input from both management and educationalists; clinical staff alone do not have the resources, particularly in the present climate. The dissemination of knowledge about models has occurred mostly through qualified staff attending post-basic professional development courses such as the University of London Diploma and part-time nursing degrees. Nursing has a professional responsibility to educate itself, and this process includes keeping abreast of model development. Thus, tutors and managers must keep up with clinical nurses in the field of professional development.

For a unit team to implement a model they need information about the various models in order that they can choose one that fits their philosophy, and they need the time and encouragement to discuss the relevant issues as well as the freedom to make any changes in working practice that are necessary. This demonstrates the importance of educational and managerial input, as the tutors can facilitate learning about models while it is the manager's responsibility to encourage and provide the necessary resources such as time. Meetings might not all take place during shift hours and the very fact that staff are prepared to meet and discuss their plans in their own time should act as a spur to management to spare no effort in helping clinical staff develop their practice.

Educationalists and managers can benefit from supporting clinical staff in this way. For the tutors it offers a way of overcoming the criticism that they teach in a vacuum and never work in the real world, hence the yawning theory–practice gap. By helping staff to learn about a model and being involved in its development in a real clinical situation, tutorial staff are bringing together theory and practice in a way that facilitates the requirements of good practice and also the teaching of models as part of the Project 2000 curriculum.

For the manager, developing a happy nursing team with a high degree of job satisfaction and commitment to their work must always be a prime goal. The sort of project outlined here could achieve that goal by allowing clinical nurses to develop their own practice in their own way. In such a situation staff recruitment and retention could become a problem of the past along with high absenteeism rates and low morale.

The manager still has budgets to contend with and must be able to show that quality care is also cost-effective care. However, when the cost of treating avoidable complications such as pressure sores and wound infections is added to the cost of hiring temporary agency staff when there are high sickness rates, it becomes apparent that quality nursing care can be cost-effective.

The involvement of managerial and educational staff is therefore essential for the successful management of the major changes involved in introducing a nursing model. It would be beneficial to create some sort of forum within a health authority where staff from different clinical areas could meet and discuss their progress in model development. In this way mutual support could develop, solutions to problems could be shared and comparisons made between the different models under development in the district. The movement of nursing education towards higher education might lead to staff from these areas being brought in to assist NHS staff in their model development. First-hand experience of model implementation should be welcomed by nurses working in academic departments as it offers priceless opportunities for the development of both nursing theory and practice.

So far we have seen that for change to be successful it must come from within. The decision to introduce a model must be taken collectively by the clinical team, as must decisions about nursing philosophy and finally the actual choice of model itself. Before actually introducing the model the educational and managerial input that went into selecting the model must continue to allow staff to develop their knowledge base and to ensure a smooth change to new working practices. Staff have to become comfortable with the model and to have a common shared understanding of what is being attempted; this requires learning about the model. In addition there needs to be a careful review of what working practices will have to change, such as patient allocation becoming primary nursing.

An old adage in education is that it is not what is taught that counts, but what is learnt. It may seem a good idea to organize a series of lectures on Model X, but that is of limited value if little is learnt about how to apply the model in practice. An introductory lecture might serve to map out the ground, and readings from the literature will also be useful, but there is no substitute for active learning.

Staff need, therefore, to draw up an education programme to ensure that everybody has had the chance to learn how to use the model in practice. This means working in small tutorial groups, discussing how different terms and concepts within the model should be interpreted. Role playing is a valuable learning tool, with members of the team taking it in turns to play a patient while colleagues carry out an assessment and try to draw up a care plan based on the model. The finished care plan can then be reviewed by the 'patient' and feedback given to the planners. Observers may comment also. An innovative gaming approach to model development has been described by Hoon (1986) in which a board game may be developed to show how differing models might affect various patients. These sorts of methods constitute an active learning approach which can be recommended as it forms the basis for teaching models of nursing used by the authors of this book.

The emphasis in this learning period before model introduction should be on practical usage and ensuring that all staff have a common understanding of how the model will be used. Brainstorming sessions to suggest ways of adapting the model to the clinical area and also to agree documentation would be an integral part of this learning process. Group activity along these lines should help foster a feeling of team spirit and a sense that this model actually belongs to the staff who are going to work with it because they have all helped to put the project together. The views of all members of the nursing team should be given equal weight — there is nothing better than perceived hierarchies for destroying team spirit.

Once the appropriate changes in nursing systems have been made and the staff have a working knowledge, then it is time to launch the

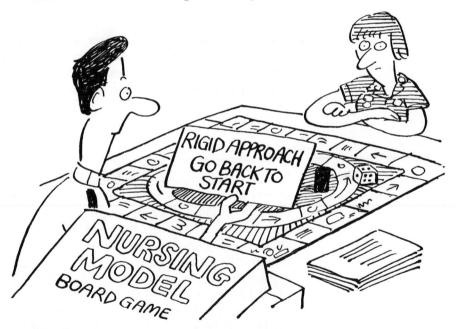

model in practice. It will not be plain sailing and nobody should expect it to be so; what matters is that mistakes are turned into positive learning experiences. Feedback should be sought at regular intervals from all the staff to allow the development and modification of the model in practice (inductive reasoning, p. 7), while quality assurance monitoring is a desirable parallel development.

In an ideal world, a quality assurance programme would be in place pre- and post-introduction of the model to see whether it made any significant difference to the standards of care or to the way the staff felt about their work. Being realistic, it would probably absorb all the energies of the staff just to introduce the model and the new systems

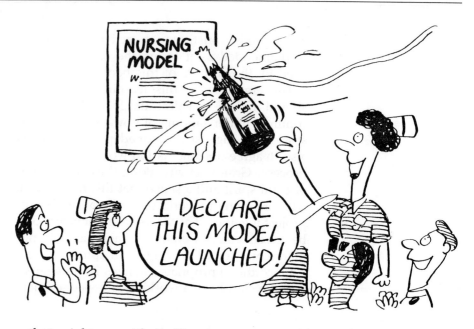

that might go with it. However, opportunities such as these almost demand that nurse researchers devote their energies to such investigations, for this represents innovative and creative nursing that is pushing at the very limits of the profession as we know it today.

Summary   In this chapter we have estabished that models of nursing really do matter because they represent a way of defining exactly what it is we mean by nursing, thereby mapping out the terrain for both education and practice. However, they are at present only collections of ideas about nursing, not theories in the strict scientific sense. In that form, though, they offer us a wonderful opportunity to be creative, for their application allows nurses to develop and refine these ideas in the light of experience gained in the clinical field.

The introduction of a model should be a bottom-up exercise being led by clinical staff with educational and management support. The unit team together with patients need to identify a broad philosophy of care and only then select a model to fit that philosophy. They should not be afraid to borrow bits from other models if appropriate. Introduction of a model needs careful preparation and education of all the staff involved, and patients where appropriate. Evaluation and feedback to modify the model are key points once it has been implemented. Finally, there is no place for a dogmatic single-model approach; students of nursing and care settings should be familiar with several differing models as such a range of care options is essential to reflect the variety in care needs of the patient population.

References

Aggleton PR & Chalmers H (1987) Models of nursing, nursing practice and nurse education. *Journal of Advanced Nursing*, **12**, 573–581.

Benner P (1984) *From Novice to Expert*. Menlo Park, Calif.: Addison Wesley.

Botha E (1989) Theory development in perspective: the role of conceptual frameworks and models in theory development. *Journal of Advanced Nursing*, **14**, 49–55.

Faucett J, Ellis V, Underwood P, Naqvi A & Wilson D (1990) The effect of Orem's self care model in a nursing home setting. *Journal of Advanced Nursing*, **15**, 659–666.

Field PA (1987) The impact of nursing theory on the clinical decision making process. *Journal of Advanced Nursing*, **12**, 563–571.

Hammersley M & Atkinson P (1983) *Ethnography: Principles in Practice*. London: Tavistock Publications.

Hardy LK (1986) Identifying the place of theoretical frameworks in an evolving discipline. *Journal of Advanced Nursing*, **11**, 103–107.

Hoon E (1986) Game playing: a way to look at nursing models. *Journal of Advanced Nursing*, **11**, 421–427.

Hunt M (1987) The process of translating research findings into nursing practice. *Journal of Advanced Nursing*, **12**, 101–110.

King I (1981) *A Theory for Nursing*, New York: Wiley.

Kristjanson LJ & Tamblyn R (1987) A model to guide development and application of multiple nursing theories. *Journal of Advanced Nursing*, **12**, 523–529.

Laughlin M (1988) Modelled, muddled and befuddled. *Nursing Times*, **84**(4), 30–31.

Lister P (1987) The misunderstood model. *Nursing Times*, **83**(4), 40–42.

Luker K (1988) Do models work? *Nursing Times*, **84**(5), 27–29.

Morales-Mann E & Logan M (1990) Implementing Roy's Model: challenges for educators. *Journal of Advanced Nursing*, **15**, 142–147.

Orem D (1985) *Nursing; Concepts of Practice*. New York: McGraw Hill.

Orlando I (1961) *The Dynamic Nurse Patient Relationship*. New York: GP Putnam.

Peplau H (1952) *Interpersonal Relationships in Nursing*. New York: GP Putnam.

Peters TJ & Waterman RH (1982) *In Search of Excellence*. New York: Harper & Row.

Pollit D & Hungler B (1985) *Nursing Research*. Philadelphia: Lippincott.

Riehl JP (1980) The Riehl Interaction Model. In Riehl JP & Roy C (eds) *Conceptual Models for Nursing Practice*. Norwalk, Conn.: Appleton Century Crofts.

Roy C (1984) *Introduction to Nursing; An Adaptation Model*. Englewood Cliffs: Prentice-Hall.

Rourke A (1990) Professional labelling. *Nursing Standard*, **4**(42), 36–39.

Torres G (1986) *Theoretical Foundations of Nursing*. Norwalk, Conn.: Appleton Century Crofts.

Walsh M & Ford P (1989) *Nursing Rituals; Research and Rational Actions*. Oxford: Heinemann.

Wright S (1986) *Building and Using a Model of Nursing*. London: Edward Arnold.

2 USING A MODEL

Introduction

Models must be more than just academic exercises, they should be capable of use in the practical situation if they are to be of value. To facilitate practical usage it is necessary to review the way that care is planned and also the way the systems used to deliver that care are organized.

Care planning

Care was always planned long before the phrase 'nursing process' was coined; what has changed is the method of planning. In the traditional system of nursing, care was planned around tasks, with the nurse in charge allocating to each nurse a series of jobs. The planning of this care was then documented in the bath book, bowel book, dressings book, etc., and when the tasks had been completed this would be noted in the kardex as a record of care given. Nurses have therefore always planned care, documented their plans and recorded the results of carrying out their care.

There is nothing new, therefore, in the nursing process requiring nurses to plan, write down their plans and evaluate their care, it is something we have always done. The fundamental difference, however, is that the focus of care has changed from tasks to the patient, which has required nurses to consider the whole patient as a person and not just another wound that needs dressing or another section of constipated bowel that needs unblocking.

All the much-maligned nursing process is trying to do is to get the nurse to consider the whole patient and adopt a rational, problem-solving approach to planning care for that whole person, rather than seeing the patient as just another name in a list of people to be bathed or toileted. This of course means the nurse must start thinking and working things out from first principles rather than just following orders, and that is not so easy.

Following orders is one way of avoiding stress, a mechanism that

Chapman (1983) argues leads to the perpetuation of much mindless ritual in nursing. Walsh and Ford (1989) agree with Chapman and point out that the traditional nurse training with its emphasis on getting tasks done and its lack of a questioning approach compounds the problem of getting nurses to think for themselves. There are also history and tradition hanging round nursing's neck like giant millstones, the history of female subservience and the tradition of obeying male, medical dominance. Given these powerful social forces acting on nurses, it is not surprising that the transition to a free-thinking, problem-solving approach has not been easy.

However, an individualized care planning approach is precisely what is required by models of nursing with their emphasis on the patient as a whole individual who is at the focus of nursing care. Whether a nursing model is based around helping a patient attain developmental goals, integrating and balancing the various physical and psychosocial systems of life or achieving an understanding of how roles and self-perception affect health, either way it is the whole individual that is involved. Such a coherent view of the individual person cannot be broken down into physical bits with a different nurse responsible for each. The Mona Lisa could have been painted if her arms had been painted by one artist, her eyes by somebody else and her smile by the 'smile artist', but would it have been the Mona Lisa of Leonardo Da Vinci? Just as great works of art and literature come from the integrated approach of one person, so caring for patients is best carried out in this integrated holistic fashion.

Nursing must therefore move away from its task-centred tradition and develop an individualistic care planning approach that requires thought, analysis and creativity on the part of the nurse. In other words, it requires the use of the nursing process with an open-minded approach. In the previous chapter the hostility and cynicism that surrounds this topic were explored; however, now is the time to be positive and creative if we are to make progress. Perhaps it is time for an amnesty on the nursing process and a fresh start. It will be worthwhile, therefore, to see how the familiar stages of care planning are influenced by nursing models.

Assessment   Unfortunately, patient assessment is often poorly carried out. It is frequently lumped together with admission, to the point now that many wards talk of admitting rather than assessing a new patient. If it is seen as a chore to be done on admission, there will be little chance of ongoing assessment, yet this is vital to monitor the success of care and to detect the emergence of new problems. When mixed up with the admission procedure, assessment tends to become delegated to a junior member of staff and interpreted as little more than a form-filling procedure for the kardex. Much vital information is missed and what is recorded lies unused in the care plan, ignored and forgotten.

Assessment must be seen as the beginning of nursing care and more than just a part of the admission procedure. Without a thorough assessment individualized nursing care cannot exist, as there is no knowledge base about the patient from which to identify problems and plan care. Care becomes standardized, routinized and impersonal as all patients are treated much the same with only their medical diagnosis having any influence on care. Nursing a patient recovering from a colostomy operation is clearly very different from nursing someone who has had a prostatectomy, but no two ostomy patients are the same either as they are unique people entitled to care tailored to their individuality. The only effective way this care can be delivered is if the nursing assessment has clearly established the individuality of the patient.

Different models have varying approaches to care and consequently seek to discover different types of knowledge about the patient and family. The nursing assessment therefore must reflect the model's philosophy. In practice the authors of models usually suggest detailed assessment schedules, which can be very helpful. An assessment schedule derived from a model has the strength of being as comprehensive as possible because the author will have thought a great deal about the assessment and tried to ensure that the nurse has the logical and consistent framework of knowledge necessary to plan care consistent with the model.

However, some notes of caution are needed. Firstly, the nurse must see the assessment form as a tool which will enable staff to make the model work, it is not just another form-filling, box-ticking exercise. Assessment must therefore reflect the aspirations of the model. If, for example, the nurse is using Orem's self-care model and discovers that the patient has a self-care deficit in being unable to maintain continence, the assessment should not stop at ticking a box on a form. Gentle and tactful probing is necessary to find out whether this problem is associated with other events or time of the day, how frequently it occurs, what measures the patient takes to deal with the problem, whether others know of the problem and if so how they help, and of course how the patient personally feels about the continence difficulties. In this way the nurse is using the self-care concept to probe and discover as much as possible about how this continence problem affects the whole life of the patient, how the patient sees the problem and how the patient attempts to manage their self care, rather than stopping at the simple statement that the patient cannot maintain self-care in terms of continence. Such an approach is consistent with the need to explore the patient's problems from varying points of view using interactionist, systems and developmental perspectives (p. 9).

The second note of caution concerns jargon. If staff find the sorts of words used by the author of a model difficult to understand, then they should consider alternative wordings that are perhaps closer to commonly used English. The purpose of words is to convey rather than obscure meaning; if they fail to convey meaning they are of no value. Nurses should not be afraid, therefore, to change the language of models, including the key words used in an assessment schedule, as long as they retain the meaning. For example, Orem's 'self-care deficit' could be changed into 'self-care problem' or Roy's 'focal stimuli' might translate into 'principal cause of problem'.

A model-based assessment schedule should be only a tool in the hands of the assessor, it must not take over and rigidly determine the course of the assessment. The nurse must be free to explore detailed areas with patients that do not have headings on the assessment plan. It may well be that patients want to talk about things that do not neatly dovetail with the headings devised by the author of a model! Rather than try to force these areas into the assessment document artificially, it is better to leave a blank space for 'other issues' which might be raised in this way. (See Chapter 5 for a discussion of how this may be applied to community care.) .

After using a model for some time it might be possible to go back over a series of patient assessments and see whether any recurring themes tend to crop up under 'other issues'. In this way the assessment schedule could be modified to incorporate areas that the model has overlooked, despite the author's attempts to make it comprehensive. For example, the nurse may note that patients' views of their illnesses are unrealistic or that many patients seem lacking in knowledge about their condition. As a result the assessment could be modified by borrowing from the interactionist approach to include a section which explored the patient's views of their illness in some detail. Alternatively, to use a more concrete example, if Roy's model were used on a surgical ward, staff might notice that there was no obvious heading under which to record essential information about a patient's wound or ability to maintain personal hygiene, and so modify the original assessment tool in this way. This is just one example of the way models can be developed and improved in practice (see p. 7).

There will be other situations when a thorough and comprehensive assessment is either not possible or is inappropriate and the nurse must recognize this possibility. Consider the patient brought to the A&E unit with multiple trauma after a road accident, or the patient who is having day surgery. In the former case, assessment should focus on life-threatening areas such as the ABC of resuscitation, pain and fear, while in the latter case it may be very interesting to know the patient's hobbies, but of little relevance if the person is going to have surgery and be sent home all in the same day.

The message here is that just because a model has defined an area as worthy of assessment, it does not necessarily have to be assessed if the patient's condition indicates otherwise. Flexibility of thought and a little bit of plain common sense should ensure that the nurse only fills in the parts of the assessment document that are needed. This also helps deal with the criticism that the nursing process wastes time due to form filling; it is the nurse who often wastes time by recording information that is not needed. Assessment is an on-going process, and parts of the assessment schedule can be completed later as part of the reassessment process and as the patient's condition allows.

We have suggested that some thought about the depth of the assessment is needed. It is essential also for the nurse to think about how the assessment is carried out if the maximum amount of useful information is to be gathered. Any model's assessment schedule is only a tool, and like a saw or drill it has to be used correctly to get the best results that it is capable of. The following observations apply to assessment, whatever the model used.

The social sciences have taught us that first impressions really do count in human interactions (Hilgard *et al.*, 1987). This has two significant implications for a nurse assessing a patient, the first of which is that we should be careful how we approach the situation. An offhand manner or an initial appearance of disorganization (e.g. calling the patient the wrong name) may create an unfortunate impression that will last for days with the patient. Conversely, the nurse should beware his or her own first impression of the patient who may be very anxious and worried by their strange surroundings, leading to abnormal behaviour as a result of this stress.

The need for privacy and good communication skills in assessment was emphasized by McFarlane and Castledine (1982) and has been recognized by most authors since. The use of a clipboard and official-looking papers with the nurse scribbling away furiously in between stereotyped questions is not the way to make the patient relax and disclose what might be very sensitive and embarrassing information. It is worth considering a cultural point here, most models are American in origin and American society is on the whole more open than British. Is it possible that some models might seek information that American citizens might volunteer more readily than the more reserved British? This would seem an area worthy of research if models developed in the USA are to be used in the UK.

Nursing models by their innovative and holistic nature may be exploring personal areas which nurses using the task-centred, medical model approach to nursing have traditionally stayed away from. When the cultural point raised in the preceding paragraph is taken into account also, the importance of privacy, sensitivity and good communication becomes apparent in a model-based assessment.

There seems little point in repeating questions which seek information that is readily available from admission documents and case notes, although such information can be stated to the patient who may then be asked to confirm that it is correct. In this way time is saved, the patient is not subjected to the annoying experience of having the same questions repeatedly asked, and the nurse demonstrates knowledge of and interest in the patient. It is always good policy to begin an assessment interview in this non-threatening factual way and it allows the patient to correct any inaccuracies such as a change of address or work. In this way the ice is broken and the patient can start to relax.

Patients' privacy must be respected at all times and if they show a reluctance to talk about an aspect of their health the nurse should not at this stage continue to push the matter. At a later time when the patient has gained more confidence, they may respond to a gentle prompt such as "When we talked a couple of days ago you seemed a little unhappy at talking about . . . ". The assessment is not a one-off event, but rather an ongoing process.

It is important for nurses who are going to work with models that they acquire good communication skills that will allow them to gently probe into sensitive areas that nursing has previously avoided. Roy's adaptation model, for example, seeks to discover a great deal about a person's self-concept and role function. Consider a woman who has been admitted for mastectomy and how she perceives herself and her role as both a woman and a sexual partner; assessment here requires more than a couple of questions with yes/no answers that allow the nurse to tick a couple of boxes.

The emphasis on introducing the social sciences into Project 2000 education is well placed for a variety of reasons, not least of which is the hope that it might considerably improve nurses' communication and assessment skills.

A model of nursing can therefore shape and guide the assessment process to ensure that data relevant to the person's individual care within the model's framework is collected. The nurse must also have an open mind and be aware of areas the patient wishes to discuss that are not detailed by the model assessment document. Good communication skills are essential to explore sensitive and personal areas with the patient.

Problems

The patient assessment should provide the nurse with sufficient information to begin working out the patient's problems. Regardless of the model used, some key points bear reiteration at this stage.

The problems identified must be patient centred (Marriner, 1979) and not nursing problems. A mistake commonly made is to write statements such as 'Patient needs enema' under the problem heading on a care plan. That is a nursing intervention, the organization of which might well be a problem; however, the patient's problem is (presumably) that he or she has not had a bowel movement for several days.

The fact that the problem is patient centred means that technical medical labels should be avoided. The nurse should try to imagine how the patient sees their problem, or better still, ask the patient to describe the problem. For example, a patient who has peripheral vascular disease (PVD) may be unable to walk more than 50 yards without developing severe calf pain. The *patient's* problem is 'severe pain on walking more than 50 yards', not a statement such as 'intermittent claudication' or 'PVD', neither of which will mean anything to the patient.

Problems also need to be prioritized in order that the most important are seen to first. Marriner (1979) suggested using Maslow's familiar Hierarchy of Needs as one method of prioritization, starting with physiological problems before moving on to problems associated with safety, love, esteem and self-actualization in that order. Within the physiological area it would seem prudent to ensure that problems relating to the basic ABC of resuscitation (Airway, Breathing, Circulation) come first, followed by pain as the next highest priority.

It is possible, however, that the patient may see problem priorities very differently from the nursing staff. This may be resolved by giving information to help a middle-aged man understand why the nurse is so insistent on getting him out of bed the morning after his operation and performing deep breathing exercises when all he wants to do is lie in bed and go to sleep.

This example illustrates the importance of potential problems, for here it is extremely unlikely that the patient will understand the nursing care being carried out. The patient's priority might be the actual problem of feeling awful and just wanting to be left alone as a result, while the nurse's priority is the potential problem of respiratory and vascular complications, hence the active interventions. Wherever there are potential and actual problems, it is probable that priorities will differ between patient and nurse, although they can also differ when actual problems alone are considered. A noisy phone can be far more of a problem to a patient at night than the nurse could ever imagine! This raises the interesting point of what input night staff should have into planning care. Patients may have problems that are specific to night-time and therefore most appropriately dealt with by night staff. The nursing process does not stop at 9 p.m.

Having made these general remarks about problems, it is necessary to look at how models affect this stage of the care planning process. A model reflects a definite philosophy of care and therefore the model will seek to define problems in such a way as to be consistent with its philosophy. The nurse should try to use the language of the model in stating problems, for this will reflect the ideas inherent in the model. When working with Orem, for example, this means seeing problems in terms of the inability to practice self-care, while with Roper's model a patient problem can be seen as an inability to perform some activity of daily living.

Is it possible that an aspect of human behaviour might be defined as a problem by one model but not by another? Given the different perspectives and conceptual frameworks employed by the authors of various models, this possibility raises itself and could be a source of significant difficulty in model development. If by simply changing from one model to another a patient's problem ceases to exist, then might not some doubt be cast on the validity of at least one of the two models in question, or do we accept that all things are relative and that, in the absence of absolute truth, differing models of nursing may well lead to different patient problems being identified?

Perhaps one way forward is to set up a study which will analyse a sample of patients using a series of models. To some extent, problems will vary as the assessment tool itself varies, but is there a limit in the amount of variation that is tolerable, beyond which nurses may start questioning the model itself and asking whether this is an appropriate model to use for this patient? Certainly, if problems emerge and disappear simply by changing models then the choice of model could play a major part in the nursing care received by any patient.

One method of setting up a study might be to have one or two researchers role play a series of patients while nurses assess them independently with different models to arrive at problem statements (and goals and interventions). Alternatively, a panel of 'experts' might independently assess patient profiles drawn from real patients using differing models. It would be very interesting to see what variation if any in problems and care arose from such an exercise.

An interesting piece of research by Faucett *et al.* (1990) has shed some light on this area. These researchers studied two comparable 50-bed continuing care wards in a US veterans administration nursing-home care unit. In one ward a 2½-year period of implementation of the Orem self-care model had taken place while the other ward had remained with the traditional nursing methods of the institution. The study took place in the final 6 months of this implementation period.

The researchers carried out a survey of patient care plans looking to see what differences in patient problems were identified and also interviewed the staff of the two units. They found that the documentation showed little significant differences, in that staff on both wards tended to identify the same problems with the same frequency and carry out the same interventions.

Interviewing showed that nurses on the ward using Orem showed more comprehensiveness in their approach to assessment and also had a greater degree of internal consistency in how they assessed patients. The use of the model, therefore, seemed to lead to a more integrated view of the patient, reflected in this more comprehensive approach. The latter point about internal consistency is relevant to the argument that models might improve nursing care by providing a framework to facilitate patterning of information as this seems to have happened here (p. 16). The nurses using Orem also showed a greater interest in securing patient participation in the process of goal setting and were much more aware of the importance of the patient being actively involved in care.

In an attempt to understand why there appeared to be this paradox that nurses using the Orem model at interview showed a very different approach to care which was not reflected in the written care plans, the researchers constructed six patient vignettes from the data available to them. These were summarized versions of patient case histories and their nursing care. These vignettes were then sent to four independent expert assessors to see if they could tell which patients were on the traditional control ward and which the experimental Orem ward. The experts agreed unanimously and correctly on four vignettes but were split on the remaining two, one of which was from the control ward and one the experimental.

This suggests that it was possible to detect from the way care plans overall were written a difference between the ward using the Orem model and the traditional model. However, in terms of problem statements and nursing interventions for real patients the researchers conclude that the overall effects of the institution's policies and procedures has dominated the nursing documentation to such an extent that what is written about these aspects of care makes it impossible to differentiate between the Orem ward and traditional ward. This is despite clear differences in how the nurses talk about assessing their patients, goal setting and the involvement of patients in care.

Researchers are familiar with the differences between what people say, write and actually do. This study appears to have run into this problem and further direct observational study of the nursing care carried out would help resolve the argument about whether implementing a model of nursing makes any difference. Researchers and clinicians need to tackle this fundamental problem of measuring changes in nursing care before meaningful research can be carried out on the effects of nursing models in practice.

In the preceding section, models were identified as taking the nursing assessment into unfamiliar territory. It follows from this that the sorts of problems that may be identified may also be unfamiliar to nurses. This has a clear knock-on effect for the rest of the care plan in terms of setting goals and deciding upon interventions. The use of models may lead British nurses into uncharted waters. This is no reason for not using them, but rather should serve as a stimulus for professional development in acquiring new skills to deal with the sorts of problems that have not previously been identified in traditional practice.

This challenge can be partly met by the Project 2000 reforms, which are all about producing a new sort of nurse. Anybody who thinks they are simply changing the way nurses obtain their qualification has a very blinkered view and is certainly in for a rude awakening once

Project 2000 nurses are allowed the freedom to practise. Changes to post-basic education are essential also, and it is encouraging that the UKCC are undertaking such a review at present (Casey, 1989). Finally, a plea should be entered for the development of nurse practitioners, as they too should be able to move into the new areas that might be identified by models.

Goals

Goals, like problems, should be patient centred. They are things we hope the patient will achieve, not the nurse. Writing '4 hrly obs' as a goal is a mistake, it is a nursing intervention. The relevant goal here might be 'Patient vital signs to stay within normal limits'.

This raises the question of what normal limits are and with it two more key points about goals: as far as possible they should be measurable and unambiguous. Thus, our goal statement might be better written with a qualification as follows: 'Patient vital signs to stay within normal limits, i.e. systolic BP 90–130, P 70–80, RR 12–16, T 36–37°C. Perhaps this might be better broken down into a series of separate goals depending on the condition of the patient; the limits set should also reflect the patient. Thus, they would be very different if the patient was a 6-month-old baby. Similarly, a goal statement such as 'Adequate fluid intake' is unacceptable as it is too ambiguous — it can mean different things to different people. However 'Patient will have intake of 3L fluid in 24 hours' is patient centred, measurable and unambiguous.

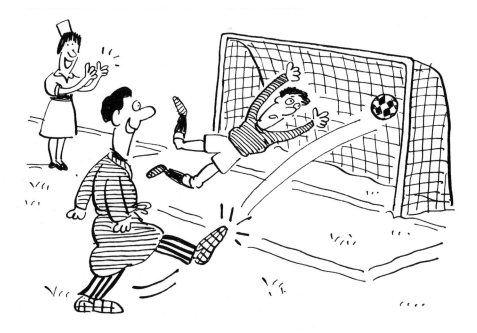

In writing this goal, the nurse has added another ingredient of goal setting — a time scale, in this case 24 hours. One of the main purposes of setting a goal is to set a standard by which we measure care, so a time limit must be set. Thus, if the nurse adds up the fluid balance chart and finds the patient only managed 2L of fluid in the 24-hour period, we know that the patient failed to achieve what was required and therefore we must ask what was wrong with the nursing care.

Goals can be set to different time scales varying from a few hours to weeks. Time scales must also be realistic. Thus, if a patient is severely overweight a goal of losing 5 kg is desirable, but unrealistic if the patient is only given 24 hours to achieve it in. Realism is the next key ingredient in goal setting. However, supposing the patient does not wish to lose weight? The weight loss goal could be written in a patient centred, measurable, unambiguous, realistic, time-limited way, but come to nought if the patient does not share the goal with the nurse. Goals should therefore be negotiated with the patient.

How will the use of models ensure that these criteria for goals are met? By attempting to place the whole patient at the focus of care, they should ensure that goals are patient centred. The emphasis placed by some models on family and significant others should also help to bring these very important people into the goal-setting process, crucial in community care settings. Other mdoels are based on the full involvement of the patient in care (e.g. King) and therefore should go even further in ensuring that patients are equal partners in goal setting.

Careful use of words in writing goals should avoid ambiguity and ensure that they are measurable in many cases. However, the use of models opens up a whole Pandora's box of unquantifiables such as fear, anxiety, self-concept and dependence. We cannot put numbers against such subjective properties, unlike a temperature reading, but that is no reason for slamming the lid shut on the box. Models and holistic care have helped liberate these aspects of our patients and we have to incorporate them into care planning.

Most patients have always had anxieties and fears. This fact has not just been recognized since models of nursing were introduced. However, nursing models do raise nurses' awareness of such subjective areas and direct their attention towards the psychological and social aspects of care in a way that the medical model never did, legitimizing them in the process.

As an example, Roy's model may allow the nurse to identify under its self-concept and role-function headings the problem that the woman undergoing mastectomy is frightened that she will no longer be sexually attractive to her husband. How does the nurse set a measurable, unambiguous goal here? Clearly any goal must be acceptable to the woman (negotiated with the patient) and might be seen as one small step along the road (short-term) to a long-term goal that the couple's sex life will return to its normal level before the surgery. For many nurses this is already unfamiliar territory. The first goal might therefore be that the man will look at his wife's operation site. However, even if this is achieved in a few days, the patient will be ready for discharge, leaving the surgical ward nurse's care plan hanging in mid-air.

This unsatisfactory example has several lessons. Firstly, when we move outside physiology, not all goals can be as neatly packaged as a fluid-intake or weight-loss goal; secondly, the nurse needs to recognize that long-term goals may be very long-term with a rather roundabout route involving a lot of shorter-term goals on the way; and thirdly, there needs to be a facility for transferring the care plan to community or specialist outpatient nursing staff to continue care directed at long-term goals. In such circumstances, attention should be given to the need to continue care along the lines of the model used in hospital, or whether a different model is now indicated. The converse is also true when a patient under care in the community is hospitalized.

In many areas of care, a goal might simply be that the patient will feel able to talk about something or will show a realistic view of their life situation when discussing a topic. Nurses in the field of mental health will be only too aware of this already, but now general nurses are coming to see goal setting in these terms also as they explore the more holistic aspects of care generated by the use of individualized care planning and models.

In conclusion, it remains to say that goals, like problems, should be worded in terms consistent with the philosophy of the model and have targets that reflect the model's view of nursing and health.

Interventions

It is crucial if a model is to be used that its philosophy should be felt in the field of practical nursing interventions. The use of a model should open up new areas in terms of patient problems and in this way influence interventions, although this brings with it the need for nurses to acquire new skills and knowledge. A model might also indicate new ways of dealing with old problems that would have been recognized with a more traditional approach.

Consider the example of a female patient who is obese and needs to lose weight. At present a nurse may advise the patient that it is healthier for her to lose 10 kg in an attempt to encourage her to do so. That of course is correct, but it is a little vague and non-specific. If the nurse was working with Roy's adaptation model, she would be familiar with ideas such as self-concept in terms of both body image and self-worth, along with role function and interdependence, i.e. how the patient relates to, and depends upon, others. Roy's model also emphasizes physiological aspects of nutrition and elimination. The nurse therefore has many more insights into human behaviour which could allow him or her to explore various strategies to help the patient lose weight other than simply saying that it is healthier.

One more example should suffice to demonstrate that the use of models can enrich nursing care. Consider an elderly male patient who has been admitted after an acute episode of heart failure. After making a recovery he will be discharged home on several different forms of medication which will continue the drug therapy he received in hospital. The traditional drug round will have ensured that (probably) he got the right medication at the right time, but it will not have taught him what the pills are for, how many to take and when, and what side-effects to look out for.

Research by Bliss (1981) showed that one admission in ten to elderly care units was due to iatrogenic, drug-related problems, i.e. the patients had to be admitted to hospital because of the effects of the drugs they were on. If patients are taught nothing about their medication prior to discharge, this is hardly surprising. However, if Orem's self-care model was in use, then the emphasis would be on teaching the patient about their medication and where possible making him responsible for self-medication in hospital. It is reasonable to say that the patient is competent to manage his medicines at home only after he has shown that he can self-medicate, under supervision, on the ward. The use of a model of nursing therefore could fundamentally change nursing practice by making patients responsible for self-medication, where able, on the ward.

The importance of cooperation and patient compliance with nursing interventions cannot be over-emphasized. If the patient refuses to carry out nurse-suggested interventions, then, whatever model of nursing is in use, nursing care will be of little value. The importance of this for nursing is shown in the fact that according to Connelly (1987) one-half of chronically ill patients fail to achieve maximum health benefit because they fail to follow health-related recommendations. As an example, Harris (Harris and Linn, 1985) has concluded that 4 out of 5 hospital days among diabetic patients were directly related to failure to follow recommended treatment, as were 50% of cases of diabetic coma. Other workers have come to similar conclusions; for example, Levy (Levy et al., 1982) found that non-compliance with treatment among chronically ill, ambulatory patients brought about more complex and expensive hospital treatment than would have been expected as well as precipitating premature hospitalization.

Nurses and nursing models must therefore address the issue of compliance with nursing (and medical) care. It must first of all be stated that in a free society the patient always has the right to say no and refuse treatment, although it is to be hoped that the decision would be an informed one with all the facts of the situation and risks available to the patient. This underlines the importance of good communication with the patient and of the nurses being prepared where necessary to be the patient's advocate.

By incorporating the elements of patient, environment, health and nursing, a valid model should also help address the problem of compliance as it is related to the patient's perception of health and the way the surrounding environment effects the patient. Non-compliance with nursing advice to give up smoking may be understood not only in terms of nicotine addiction but also the patient's view of his health and the effect he thinks smoking has on that health ('Smoking makes me cough and clears my chest'), and also whether the patient is surrounded by other smokers at home and work, and also the messages conveyed at great expense by the advertising industry that smoking is a good thing.

The problem of compliance shows that the nurse needs an interactionist dimension to any model being used. The nurse must try to understand how the patient constructs any situation if the nurse is to have the best chance of persuading the patient to comply with treatment and care which research evidence suggests will be beneficial to the patient. The patient's developmental status will also affect their ability to cooperate in treatment, whether it be the young child who simply does not understand why she has to take her medicine or the elderly widow who has given up wanting to carry on living as part of a bereavement reaction. Once again we see that different approaches to model construction (p. 9) are all relevant in deciding upon nursing interventions.

Compliance is particularly relevant in considering the care of patients with chronic illness, and in a review of these problems Connelly (1987) emphasizes the importance of self-care in compliance, going on to discuss predisposing factors such as self-concept, family and support networks and psychological status. These are key notions in the work of Orem and Roy respectively, indicating that nursing care derived from these models can tackle problems of compliance.

It will be apparent from the previous sections that use of a model will lead nursing into some new and unfamiliar territory that will involve seeing the patient in a more holistic fashion. One major change that will be noticed in using most models is that the nurse needs to spend more time talking to the patient and this must be recognized as direct nursing care, not just 'having a chat'. Managers and Sisters therefore should accept that time spent in conversation, particularly listening to a patient, is very much a part of nursing intervention as time spent bathing or dressing the patient.

The nurse may find that models start to identify environmental problems whose solutions lie beyond the boundaries of nursing at present. This is particularly true of the community nurse. This is no reason to reject models, although this may be a very frustrating situation for the community nurse to be in. Rather we must look at ways in which nursing can tackle these new problem areas and not just walk away from them. It may be that closer links with social services are needed. The nurse as patient's advocate is a role that nursing spends more time talking about than practising; perhaps models may force nurses to confront the reality of that role. In this way models can serve as a stimulus to nursing development.

On a larger scale still, perhaps some patient's problems have their origins in political decisions made by local government or even national government, e.g. the reduction in child benefits and social security reforms of the Thatcher government between 1987 and 1989. Or perhaps it is the factory down the road producing unacceptable levels of pollution. If nursing models make us recognize the political and environmental causes of some patient problems, there should be no logical reason why nursing should not go forwrd into these arenas as a legitimate part of nursing intervention.

The 1980s have witnessed a gradual increase in participation in political and social issues by the Royal College of Nursing and other health unions. This is a long-overdue development which is to be welcomed. At individual level, perhaps it is time nurses became involved in local campaigns to clean up the environment.

Models may also lead nurses to place greater emphasis on patients learning to do things for themselves. Not only do nurses need to learn what is involved in allowing and encouraging a patient self-care, but so do patients and their families. The danger is that what to the nurse appears as interventions designed to promote independence in activities of daily living (Roper) or to improve self-care ability (Orem) may look to the patient like neglect.

This underlines the need for good communication between nursing staff, patient and family in order that the patient knows what the nurse is trying to achieve. Misunderstandings which could lead to complaints can be avoided in this way.

Evaluation   The need for continual reassessment has already been emphasized, in this way, evaluation of care given can be achieved and any new problems identified. Evaluation should be consistent with the model. Thus the nurse will tend to be assessing how self-caring or independent the patient is, depending on the model in use.

Care in the less well-defined psychological areas that a model may lead into is not so easy to evaluate, as measurable goals are not so readily set (p. 34). Nursing judgements become very subjective concerning how well a patient is adapting to a change in self-concept after mastectomy for example (Roy). The nursing team would benefit from discussing patients and sharing among themselves views about why a nurse thinks patient X is making progress towards adaptation.

In this way some common standards can be developed in what is otherwise a very subjective area.

By way of an analogy, if a patient on head injury observations is to be handed from one nurse to another, they should do a set of observations together to ensure agreement on key parameters such as response to verbal stimuli. In this way any changes recorded are more likely to be real rather than simply variations in the perception of two different members of staff. If the ward team can arrive at some common understanding of what constitutes a reduction in anxiety or a more realistic world view by the patient, then evaluation of care can start to become more reliable in these very subjective areas. Differences are more likely to be real rather than a reflection of variations in the different nurses' perceptions of the progress being made.

The community nurse, however, is in a more isolated position and will tend to be the only nurse seeing a patient at any given time, compared to the ward situation where many nurses are involved simultaneously. This makes discussion within the community team more difficult, which in turn makes it all the more important that community nurses discuss the psychosocial progress all their patients make. Patterns and key signs can start to emerge which can be applied by staff to their own patients to assess progress and hence evaluate care.

Care planning and standard care plans

Nurses are often heard to say that the nursing process takes too long because of all the time spent on paperwork. We have already suggested that some of this is time wasted by the nurse recording unnecessary data. However, there is no denying that time is required for writing care plans. It must be said that properly organized and documented care can also save time, e.g. it avoids the nurse who is to do a dressing trying to find another nurse who knows what is used for the dressing and how long it is since last performed, sometimes unsuccessfully and always at a cost in time.

It is from the need to save time that the notion of standardized care plans evolved. The principle is that certain groups of patients would tend to have a common set of problems and therefore a team of nurses could plan care in advance and draw up a standard or common core care plan to which individualized aspects could be added according to the individual patient's needs.

Advantages include savings in time, the pooling of knowledge that occurs as experienced nurses work in a team to draft plans and the fact that the care plan can be a great help to inexperienced nurses. Walsh (1990) has shown how they may be used in A&E nursing, while another approach has been described by Glasper *et al.* (1987).

Standardized care plans could also be incorporated into a quality assurance exercise, as in setting goals in this way the nursing team are effectively setting standards or criteria against which the outcome of care can be evaluated. However, there is a clear danger that the very elements of individuality that models of nursing are striving to promote may be lost in this way. If standardized care plans are not preceded by a thorough assessment and the identification of individual problems which are also incorporated into care, then they degenerate into little more than a list of tasks and cannot be considered individualized patient care.

Primary nursing and the organization of care delivery

So far we have identified two elements necessary for the delivery of professional nursing in the 1990s: a rational nursing model and a system of planning individualized care. It now remains to look at the third and final component, the actual system of organizing nurses and nursing.

The traditional system was based around tasks with each nurse assigned a task to perform for all patients that shift. As we know this led to fragmentation and depersonalization of care as patients found a bewildering array of nurses coming and going performing separate tasks with no sense of continuity or order. Psychological and social aspects of care never had much chance of developing in this task-centred system. The next development came with the advent of team nursing and patient allocation. The idea was that by allocating a group of patients to a team of nurses, or a smaller group to a single nurse, care would become more holistic. Walsh and Ford (1989) have argued that in practice team nursing tends to resemble a small-scale version of task allocation, while the single nurse who has a small group of patients allocated to her or him for a shift finds it very difficult to practise holistic care because there is no continuity beyond that shift. Come the following day, responsibility has been passed on to somebody else while the nurse is given a new set of patients, again for the duration of only a shift before this game of musical chairs is repeated again and again.

This lack of continuity of care is compounded by the low standard of care planning and documentation that may be due to a lack of time or knowledge of care planning techniques. The nurse may also have a strongly negative attitude towards the subject, which inhibits good care planning. To take over responsibility for a batch of eight new patients in the morning is a daunting prospect, but when there is only a very scant written record of their problems and care, and that may be several days or even weeks out of date, then the chances of the nurse being able to practise professional individualized care start to become very slim indeed.

A model of nursing can give the nurse a framework and a philosophy to work with, but there has to be a system of nursing that permits a nurse to implement care consistently and in a way that meets the patient's individual needs as well as the need for professional accountability on the part of the nurse. This system is primary nursing.

Primary nursing is another import from the United States, but has a major contribution to make if nursing models and individualized care are to be made to work. The notion is simply that each patient has a nurse who retains overall responsibility for their care in the same way that a doctor does. This nurse, the primary nurse, should assess and plan care, delegating responsibility for the patient to colleagues or associate nurses when off duty (MacGuire, 1988).

In this way the continuity of care so sadly lacking at present from patient allocation or team nursing systems can be achieved. A model of nursing is more likely to be successful if the nurse can get to know the patient well, starting with a careful assessment, and care once planned can be carried out in accordance with that nurse's wishes (and the patient's of course!). The present fragmented system militates against much of what was said in the first part of this chapter. Assessment and reassessment to evaluate care and progress, exploring the more personal areas of the patient's life, the increasingly subjective aspects of care such as adaptation to surgery or feelings of self-worth and the sensitive settings of goals all require nurses to build relationships with patients.

The community nurse visiting the patient at home cannot help but start to get to him or her as a person, while the nurse in the field of mental illness has long realized the importance of getting to know patients and their families. Sadly, however, general hospital-based nurses have in the past often failed to get to know their patients as individuals, while current trends in throughput and staffing levels are not conducive to this process either.

Primary nursing redefines the traditional nurse–patient relationship by bringing both parties together in a completely new way. Wright and Khadim (1989) argue that it redefines the whole way we should think about nursing and goes far deeper than being simply a new fad or a way of allocating work. Such views are welcome and help to give primary nursing a measure of its significance and true worth.

Summary It is self-evident from a study of the various nursing models that careful planning, alongside treating the patient as an individual, is an essential prerequisite for their use. This indicates the need for a system of nursing that gives continuity of care that is best accomplished if one nurse is clearly identified as responsible for each patient, i.e. primary nursing. The reader wishing to introduce a nursing model will therefore need to introduce primary nursing and individualized care planning as the preferred means whereby the model is implemented. These changes amount to nothing less than a revolution in nursing care and, as history shows, successful revolution in nursing care and, as history shows, successful revolutions that last tend to come from the bottom up not from the top down. Introduction of the various changes inherent in model development should therefore proceed very much from the 'shop floor' upwards.

References

Bliss M (1981) Prescribing for the elderly. *British Medical Journal*, **283**, 203–204.

Casey N (1989) Editorial. *Nursing Standard*, **4**(6),3.

Chapman GE (1983) Ritual and rational action in hospitals. *Journal of Advanced Nursing*, **8**, 13–20.

Connelly CE (1987) Self-care and the chronically ill patient. *Nursing Clinics of North America*, **22**(3), 621–629.

Faucett J, Ellis V, Underwood P, Naqvi A & Wilson D (1990) The effect of Orem's self care model in a nursing home setting. *Journal of Advanced Nursing*, **15**, 659–666.

Glasper A, Stonehouse J & Martin L (1987) Core care plans. *Nursing Times*, **83** (March 11), 55–57.

Harris R & Linn MW (1985) Health beliefs, compliance and control of diabetes mellitus. *Southern Medical Journal*, **78**(2).

Hilgard E, Atkinson R, & Smith E (1987) *Introduction to Psychology*. New York: Harcourt Brace Jovanovich.

Levy M. Mermelstein L & Hemo D (1982) Medical admissions due to non-compliance with drug therapy. *International Journal of Clinical Pharacology, Therapeutics and Toxicology*, **20**(12).

MacGuire J (1988) I'm your nurse. *Nursing Times*, **84**(30), 32–36.

Marriner A (1979) *The Nursing Process*. St Louis: CV Mosby.

McFarlane J & Castledine G (1982) *The Practice of Nursing*. London: CV Mosby.

Walsh M (1990) *A&E Nursing: A New Approach*. Oxford: Heinemann.

Walsh M & Ford P (1989) *Nursing Rituals; Research and Rational Actions*. Oxford: Heinemann.

Wright S & Khadim A (1989) A Primary nursing; Your questions answered. *Nursing Standard*, **4**(7).

3 THE MODELS USED IN THIS BOOK

In the next section of the book, models will be critically evaluated in various fields of nursing by the process of attempting to devise assessments and care plans based upon the work of Orem, Roy, King, Roper and the FANCAP assessment scheme of Abbey. The application of these models to general adult nursing, both hospital and community, and mental health nursing will be explored.

In this chapter, a very brief outline of the salient features of the respective models will be given for reference. However, the reader is strongly recommended to use the reading list given at the end of the chapter to explore in detail both the original writings of the authors, and the various interpretations of their work that are available. It is only by reference to the original sources that the reader will come to understand the full philosophy of the model and the stance that the authors have taken in expressing their ideas. All models contain assumptions which are always open to question; again these will become apparent only by reference to the original sources.

The selection of models reflects those which are most commonly used and also those which seem most relevant to practical nursing. In developing the care plans, jargon has been avoided as far as possible and the documentation has been freely adapted from the author's ideas in a way that seems easiest to work with. Given the immature state of model development, the nurse is encouraged to consider further modifications beyond those that have been used to construct care plans here. Such work should be undertaken in the light of practical experience and also with reference to the literature in order that the nurse does not lose touch with the author's ideas.

Orem's self-care model

Orem's basic philosophy is that people strive to achieve self-care either by their own efforts or by the efforts of significant others such as friends or family. When they are unable to achieve self-care, a self-care deficit exists, which is defined as a patient problem requiring nursing intervention. The basic philosophy of nursing in this model is therefore to help the patient and family achieve self-care.

Patients may be envisaged as lying on a spectrum of self-care demand stretching from, for example, an unconscious patient being ventilated on ITU through to a diabetic person who needs advice about their injection technique. The former patient is unable to meet any of his self-care needs and requires total nursing intervention, which Orem calls a wholly compensatory nursing system. The latter patient requires only some advice from the nurse to provide for all their self-care needs; this is known as an educative supportive nursing system. Between these two extremes, nursing is said to be partially compensatory, implying that the patient can meet some but not all of their self-care needs.

Orem's model may analyse the nursing care for goals using the above framework and some writers insert a column on the care plan in which the nurse notes whether the nursing care for any goal is wholly or partly compensatory, or educative/consultative. This practice has not been followed in this book in the interest of simplifying the paperwork.

This model of nursing therefore acknowledges that patients can have a wide range of dependency and emphasizes the role of the nurse not only as a provider of care but also as an educator about health. The aim of the nurse is to help patients to move along this continuum of self-care need until they can achieve the maximum possible self-care with the nursing role ideally limited to support and advice.

The model emphasizes that self-care should be therapeutic, i.e. beneficial to health. The patient's perception of self care may not actually improve their health status, e.g. smoking may be seen as reducing stress and therefore to the patient may appear self-care. This dilemma of whose point of view is correct, the patient's or the nurse's, recurs in other models and requires the nurse to adopt an interactionist point of view in applying systems or developmental models.

Many health problems can be seen as originating in lack of knowledge or in self-neglect. The Orem model seeks to highlight these causes of ill health, and by stressing the importance of the educative supportive nursing system offers a way of tackling these problems. Hartweg (1990) has analysed Orem's model from the point of view of health promotion, defining this to mean positive action taken by a person to benefit health. This is congruent with Orem's ideas about self-care and Hartweg has shown that these ideas can be incorporated within the universal and developmental self-care aspects of Orem's model, making the model suitable for health promotion work.

The patient assessment is geared towards establishing self-care ability and self-care demand in order that deficits can be discovered. These self-care deficits, actual and potential, are then patient problems. Assessment is required under three broad areas, which are known as the universal, developmental and health deviancy self-care demands.

Universal self-care is primarily concerned with normal functioning and involves the required intake of air, water and nutrients to maintain health, and also their excretion. There has to be effective prevention of hazards to life and also there has to be a balance between rest and activity, social interaction and solitude. Finally, this social theme is developed into the concept of normalcy, meaning the human ability to function in groups and the desire to be accepted and seen as normal.

Developmental self-care partly reflects the way a person's developmental status affects their universal self-care ability. However, adult life also has various developmental milestones in the same way as childhood. These adult milestones may be seen as positive events such as marriage and childbirth or negative events such as divorce, redundancy at work or bereavement. The nurse needs to assess the person's ability to cope with these events and take into account how they will affect self-care ability in other areas.

Health deviancy self-care looks at the actions required by the person to cope specifically with illness and/or disability. They may be seen as a logical sequence starting with the ability to recognize that there is an illness problem and that medical attention is needed. The next steps involve the ability to recognize the likely effects of illness, being able to carry out medically prescribed treatments and being aware of possible side-effects of such treatments (e.g. drugs or diet). Finally, patients need to be able to adapt their self concept in line with their illness, learning to live with its effects while maximizing personal achievement and quality of life.

These basic ideas will be applied to derive an assessment schedule and to show how the self-care concept can be used as the basis for nursing care in the examples that follow in Chapters 4, 5 and 6.

The Roy adaptation model

Roy considers health to be a function of adaptation to stressors which may be physiological, psychological or social in origin. Successful adaptation may be equated with health and therefore the nurse's role becomes one of assisting the patient to adapt to the stressors to which he or she is exposed. The model is behaviourist in nature since at its core lies the question of how the patient behaves in response to the various stressors of life. These stressors are known as stimuli in the Roy model and nursing care is seen wherever possible as being directed at the stimuli, i.e. the causes of the patient's problems.

If a person is exposed to pathogenic micro-organisms but their body defence systems successfully prevent an infection developing, we may say they are healthy because they have adapted to the stressor. The stressor lay within the person's adaptation range, they were capable of dealing with it as the body had the appropriate antibodies, etc. If the micro-organism was one which the body could not deal with, e.g. a strain of influenza virus to which immunity had not developed, it could be said to lie outside the adaptation range of the body and illness, i.e. flu, results.

This principle of adaptation can be applied to psychosocial situations as well. Thus, a woman undergoing mastectomy will be exposed to many stressors in addition to the obvious physical stresses of surgery and cancer. She faces a major challenge to her self-concept of her body and worth as a person, along with her role function as a woman and as a sexual partner. This in turn affects her interdependence with others such as her husband or partner.

To assess a patient using the adaptation model it is necessary to describe the patient's behaviour and pick out those areas which show signs of a failure to adapt. Maladaptation is defined as a patient problem. The next step is to consider what is causing that behaviour, i.e. the stimulus, as this is ideally going to be the target for nursing intervention. The model suggests that the causes of problems can be analysed into three types, focal, contextual and residual stimuli.

The focal stimulus is the immediate cause of a problem, a contextual stimulus is seen as any environmental factor that may contribute to that problem, while a residual stimulus can be either a previous experience or an attitude or belief system which may also be a contributory factor. Thus, for every problem identified there should be a focal stimulus, and there may or may not be a contextual and/or residual stimulus.

Consider a patient who is in pain after surgery. That is the behaviour we have observed. The next step is to find out what is causing that pain and obviously the immediate answer is the direct effect of the surgery. This then is the focal stimulus or immediate cause of the pain. However, Roy's model urges the nurse to look further to see whether there are other causes.

The patient may be worried about some of the things going on around him or her in the ward and, as Hayward (1979) has shown, anxiety increases pain. This is an example of a contextual stimulus, an environmental factor contributing to pain. The patient may also have the belief that he or she should expect pain after surgery and so should not have asked for analgesia that could have relieved the pain. This is a belief or residual stimulus contributing to the patient's pain.

The nurse using the Roy model would do more than give post-op analgesia, he or she would also find our what the patient was anxious about and by explanation reduce anxiety and pain and also engage in patient teaching about pain relief to encourage the patient to ask for analgesia as soon as pain was felt rather than suffer in silence because of a mistaken belief.

Assessment is therefore a two-stage process. The first stage consists of describing patient behaviour and discovering how they are feeling and what they are thinking then trying to pick out problem areas. This is known as the first-level assessment, while the second stage, or second-level assessment, involves trying to discover the causes of the patient's problems identified in the first stage.

It may be argued that some stimuli are not amenable to nursing intervention; for example, in the case above, surgery is seen as the focal cause of the patient's pain yet clearly there is nothing the nurse can do about the fact that the patient has had surgery. The common-sense approach is to acknowledge that sometimes the causes of patient problems (stimuli) are not amenable to nursing intervention. However, the nurse can still do much to alleviate the effects of the stimuli, e.g. in this case give analgesia.

An alternative, more rigorous approach is that of Logan (1990), who argues that only those stimuli that are amenable to direct and independent nursing action should be included in the assessment. Independent action is defined as actions which nurses perform under their own initiative without needing consent or written instructions from others. According to this definition, giving analgesia is not an independent nursing action since it needs a doctor's written instructions in the form of a prescription on a drug chart.

The problem with Logan's approach may be illustrated by considering a patient who is vomiting after surgery. This could be due to a post-operative ileus or the side-effects of narcotic analgesia (the stimuli in Roy's language). As there is nothing the nurse can do to directly resolve the ileus, and as giving analgesia is not an independent nursing action, Logan seems to be suggesting that these should be ignored in the second-stage assessment process. The result is a patient who is vomiting yet, according to Logan's interpretation, we ignore the causes of the vomiting because they are not amenable to what she defines as independent nursing actions! In this book the more practical common-sense approach has been adopted rather than Logan's more extreme view.

To give structure to the assessment, the model suggests four different areas of behaviour that should be assessed: physiology, self-concept, role function and interdependence. Physiology is subdivided into oxygenation and circulation, fluid and electrolyte balance, nutrition, elimination, rest and activity and regulation, including body temperature, hormonal and nervous system control. Self-concept includes both physical (i.e. the body) and personal self-concept (i.e.

self worth), while role function concerns the various roles that the person undertakes in life — wife, mother, worker, etc. Interdependence describes the way the person relates to others.

The model therefore concerns itself with assessing patients' behaviour and their psychological and social processes using the four headings mentioned above, before going into an analysis of what may be causing the problem areas identified initially. Nursing interventions should be targeted where possible at the causes of the patient's problems and aiming always to help the patient adapt or cope with life.

The FANCAP assessment scheme

Strictly speaking this is not a model of nursing but rather a quick and comprehensive guide to assessment (Abbey, 1980) that can be bolted on to the nurse's own philosophy of care or used on its own in very acute situations such as A&E or ITU. The FANCAP scheme, therefore, is potentially a very useful building block for nurses constructing their own model, hence its inclusion.

The six letters in FANCAP are the initials of the key words Fluids, Aeration, Nutrition, Communication, Activity, Pain. The order has no significance, it is simply to make an easily remembered word. As an aid to assessment it is suggested that some of the headings are readily broken down into notions of in and out, e.g. fluids or nutrition.

A key idea in using the scheme is that the six headings should be interpreted in ways other than their literal meanings; this lateral thinking gives the scheme greater flexibility and scope. The sorts of parameters that should be assessed may be summarized as follows.

Fluids
In: Oral hydration, IVI.
Out: Urine, vomit, wound drainage, sweat (temperature)
Lateral: Fluidity means flowing along without friction, how well therefore does the person relate to others? Is he or she isolated, difficult to get along with or socially integrated and easy to get along with?

Aeration
In: Airway patency, breathing, (rate, effort, rhythm) skin colour if caucasian, evidence of cyanosis
Out: Expiratory wheeze, cough, sputum production, cardiac output (BP, P).
Lateral: Aeration implies ventilation of feelings, 'getting it off your chest'. Is the patient expressing/supressing emotions?

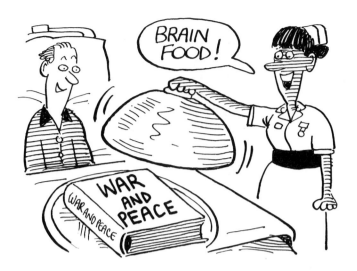

Nutrition	In:	Dietary intake.
	Out:	Bowel habit.
	Lateral:	The mind needs feeding as well as the stomach. What is the quality and quantity of mental stimulation reaching the patient?
Communication	In:	Sensory nervous system, central nervous system, ability to understand language, orientation in time and space, other neurological signs, endocrine system as an internal communication system.
	Out:	Language use, ideas expressed, non-verbal communication.
	Lateral:	Communication means a route between two separate locations, thus a wound is communication between the outside world and inside the body. Assess wounds under communication.

The final two headings do not lend themselves to the structures suggested above as it is not possible to distinguish between in and out nor is there any obvious benefit from a looser more lateral interpretation of the key words.

Activity	Rest and activity, sleep and mobility, social activity (recreation, family, etc.) and work activity should be assessed here.
Pain	Physical pain is obvious, but a looser interpretation leads to a consideration of psychological pain, i.e. fear and anxiety.

The sequence in which a patient may be assessed will vary according to the patient and their condition. Thus, in an A&E unit or ITU, aeration would be the first priority followed by pain, while in a renal care unit fluids would be the logical starting point. The nurse should make use of the various assessment tools that are available in assessing the different areas such as a pressure sore risk calculator or a pain rating scale.

The lateral thinking aspects of the scheme are often greeted initially with some scepticism, but after usage it is usually acknowledged that the scheme is made more comprehensive and sensitive by such an approach. This has been the author's experience in teaching third-year students to use FANCAP in a variety of settings.

The FANCAP scheme is deliberately left loose for nurses to adapt to their own clinical area so that it can be used on conjunction with any philosophy of care to build a nursing model suitable to that clinical area. It is a challenge to the nurse's creativity and powers of independent thinking.

The Roper activities of living model

This model is derived from the notion that humans carry out a series of everyday activities which are essential to normal functioning. The model claims that 12 such activities of living may be identified and structures nursing around this framework as follows.

(1) Maintaining a safe environment
(2) Communicating with others, both verbally and non-verbally
(3) Breathing
(4) Eating and drinking
(5) Elimination of body wastes
(6) Personal cleansing and dressing
(7) Controlling body temperature
(8) Mobilizing, both locomotion and manipulation
(9) Working and playing
(10) Expressing sexuality (appearance, relationships, etc.)
(11) Sleeping
(12) Dying

The model considers that humans exist on an independence–dependence continuum and this is reflected in each of these 12 activities of living (ALs). Thus, a person can be positioned somewhere between the two extremes for each of these 12 ALs with factors such as age and illness playing a major role in determining their exact location.

The function of nursing is seen as trying to promote maximum independence for each AL and meet the patient's needs that arise due to increasing dependence. It is important to maintain the patient's normal routine as far as possible. Where this is identified as having contributed to the patient's illness, the nurse is seen as being responsible for trying to change the patient's attitudes to be more compatible with health. The nursing role can vary from giving information to the patient through to actually carrying out an AL if the patient is unable to do it for him or herself.

The model identifies three other components of nursing besides those carried out directly in relation to these 12 ALs. These are the preventing, comforting and dependent components of nursing. Clearly, prevention of harm to the patient is a nursing responsibility which extends to encompass health education. Comforting, as its name implies, is directed at improving the physical comfort of the patient, while the dependent component of nursing involves perform- ing tasks for the patient which he/she cannot carry out unaided. There seems a lack of clarity in separating out these three components from the AL component and the authors admit that they overlap and interrelate very closely.

The use of the Roper model involves a checklist assessment of the patient's normal level of functioning under these 12 headings followed by an assessment of the patient's current levels of independence. The goal of nursing care is to restore the patient to their previous level of independence, or where this is not possible to help the patient cope with a reduced level of independence.

The reader may question the absence of any psychological or social dimension to this model and may also wonder whether human behaviour can be broken down into these 12 components. We have already seen how Rourke (1990) is very critical of the model for the way it falls into the trap of reductionism, leading to a dehumanizing process. The whole person dissolves into these 12 fragments, each of which is viewed from the negative point of view of a failure to achieve.

Why 12? Why not 10 or 15? What evidence is there to support the claim that these 12 headings represent a comprehensive and definitive view of human behaviour? Self-concept and self-worth, the patient's view of things, attitudes and beliefs spring to mind as topics not covered in this rather simplistic approach to assessment. Questions can be raised about how emotions and fears, anxiety and stress can be assessed and the problems arising from these psychological com- ponents of the human condition accounted for. There are also the effects of family, environment, housing conditions, poverty and unemployment to be accounted for.

Although the philosophy of promoting independence is one which many nurses can agree with, the above analysis suggests that the Roper model is open to significant criticism. In the following sections we will see how it stands up to these criticisms when tested against some theoretical, but representative, patients, along with the other models outlined so far.

References

Abbey J (1980) The FANCAP assessment scheme, in Riehl JP & Roy C (eds) *Conceptual Models for Nursing Practice.* Norwalk, Conn.: Appleton–Century Crofts.

Hartweg DL (1990) Health promotion self-care within Orem's general theory of nursing. *Journal of Advanced Nursing,* **15,** 35–41.

Hayward J (1979) *Information: A prescription against pain.* London: Royal College of Nursing.

Logan M (1990) The Roy Adaptation Model: are nursing diagnoses amenable to independent nurse functions? *Journal of Advanced Nursing,* **15,** 468–470.

Rourke A (1990) Professional labelling. *Nursing Standard,* **4**(42)**,** 36–39.

Bibliography

Aggleton PJ & Chalmers H (1986) *Nursing Models and the Nursing Process.* Basingstoke: Macmillan.

Orem D (1985) *Nursing: Concepts of Practice.* New York: McGraw Hill.

Roper N, Logan WW & Tierney A (1985) *The Elements of Nursing.* Edinburgh: Churchill Livingstone.

Roy C (1984) *Introduction to Nursing: An Adaptation Model.* Englewood Cliffs: Prentice–Hall.

Vaughan B & Pearson A (1986) *Nursing Models for Practice.* Oxford: Heinemann.

4 MODELS IN ADULT HOSPITAL-BASED CARE

This chapter aims to explore the requirements and ideal characteristics of a model of nursing suitable for the care of adults in a general hospital setting. These ideals will be tested by using representative patient assessments and care plans based on the Roy, Orem and Roper models along with the FANCAP assessment scheme. It is hoped that the reader will benefit by seeing how to apply these theoretical models in practice and also it will be interesting to see how effectively the models meet the criteria set out at the start of the chapter.

Ideal model characteristics

This section is not meant as a definitive list of characteristics essential for a model — it cannot be, as different nurses will have different points of view about nursing and patient priorities. However, the sort of issues raised here might usefully serve as a basis for discussion, or a starting point, when staff are considering models of nursing and what might best fit their own philosophy of care.

The whole thrust of nursing in the last decade has been directed towards seeing the patient as an integrated, individual human being rather than as a piece of malfunctioning anatomy. The patient is a person not 'the mastectomy in bed 3' or 'the man with the leg'. This means that any model of nursing must take into account the patient's psychological and social functioning as well as as anatomy and physiology.

Hospitalization is a very stressful event, carrying with it the threats of radical change to the person's body and the way it works or even the possibility of death. The whole network of social roles that have evolved over a lifetime are disrupted, e.g. roles of worker, parent, spouse or lover, possibly permanently by the hospital experience and its aftermath. The person's very existence may be threatened and their independence removed. In the light of these assaults on a person's psyche, it is evident that nursing care cannot ignore the psychological or closely related social aspects of a patient.

It is possible that the interplay of social and psychological factors was responsible for the patient's illness in the first place. How else can we explain the findings of the by now classic report *Inequalities in Health* (Black, Townsend *et al.*, 1981)? This major piece of work showed that for most forms of illness and trauma, mortality and morbidity were closely linked to social class — the poorer a person was the more likely they were to suffer or die from any given disease. Much work has been done since the publication of *Inequalities in Health* that suggests this differential has persisted throughout the 1980s (Whitehead, 1987).

Social and environmental factors are a major component of illness and need to be considered not only in relation to causation, but also when planning discharge, for the patient will return to the same sort of environment that contributed to their illness in the first place.

A model of nursing therefore needs to allow the nurse to assess the role played by social and environmental factors in causing the patient's health problems. It should make it possible to explore the patient's anxieties and fears while in hospital and how they feel about the future after discharge. The likely social setting into which the patient will be discharged should feature in the model together with the effects this may have on the patient's progress both in hospital and subsequently. Insights into the patient's feelings and emotions together with his or her family and social networks must become apparent from the model if the nurse is to achieve the aim of providing integrated, individualized care for the whole patient. The alternative is to resort to the medical model of concentrating only on the malfunctioning piece of anatomy.

Although the psychosocial aspects of care have been emphasized, the nurse must not lose sight of the physiological aspects either. The model should be sensitive to immediate life-threatening problems, to pain, and other essential aspects of bodily function.

The assessment scheme should therefore commence with the 'ABC of resuscitation' priorities of airway, breathing and circulation. The patient's respiratory and cardiovascular status are normally the highest priority for nursing assessment, followed by pain. The early discharge policy being pursued over the last few years coupled with the changing demographic profile of the general population has meant that the hospital population has become increasingly dependent and frail. Assessment of mobility is therefore essential if a whole host of potential problems related to immobility are to be avoided. Other key areas such as fluid balance and nutrition, along with personal hygiene and wound care, must also feature prominently in the assessment if problems relating to these areas are to be detected or, better still, prevented.

The reality of many hospitals today is a very rapid turnover of patients leading to discharge becoming ever sooner. The hard-pressed community services, however, cannot provide the level of care that the hospital can. This not only requires the nurse to have an increased awareness of social factors (as discussed above) but it also emphasizes the need for hospital nursing care increasingly to prepare the patient for self-care at home. Patients need more knowledge about areas such as managing their diet or medication, caring for wounds or carrying out physiotherapy after discharge.

The traditional nursing role of acting for the patient is no longer adequate for the patient's needs. Early-discharge policies require nurses to promote independence and self-care while the patient is in the supervised environment of the ward. Patients should be able to show that they are technically competent to perform whatever tasks are required and have the necessary understanding of what is involved before they can be safely discharged. The model of nursing in use therefore should lay emphasis on the nurse teaching the patient and/or family to be self-caring. A health education, patient teaching approach to nursing should be a major constituent of such a model. This would reflect a greater awareness of nursing being involved in the active promotion of health, rather than an exclusive focus on caring for the ill.

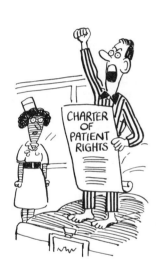

The self-care approach leads the nurse into negotiation with the patient, which in turn results in the realization that the patient also has a point of view. Nurses cannot plan care that ignores the patient's wishes and perceptions. The basic human rights of patients dictate that they must consent to the care being carried out and that consent should be informed consent. Nurses must explain not only what they are doing but why and seek the patient's approval. In that way patient cooperation is much more likely, leading to the likelihood that care will be more effective.

It is possible that a patient's apparent lack of cooperation simply stems from a deeply held, but erroneous, belief. Areas such as diet or sexual behaviour abound with such beliefs. Only when the nurse has discovered what the patient believes can his or her behaviour be put in context and more fully understood. Consider the following real example of a 55-year-old male surgical patient who continued to smoke 20 cigarettes a day despite every exhortation to the contrary pre- and post-operatively because he believed this was good for him. The reason he gave was that it allowed him to 'Have a good cough and bring up all that phlegm'. Seen from that point of view there is logic to his actions and, given that insight, the nurse now has a more realistic chance of persuading him to give up or at least reduce the smoking. The nurse might do well to try seeing a situation from the patient's perspective, things may not seem so illogical that way!

The model of nursing chosen therefore needs to be able to recognize the patient's point of view and if possible, explore beliefs and attitudes held about areas relevant to health.

The demographic changes referred to earlier are reflected in the increasing number of elderly hospital patients. The elderly have different needs from the young and middle-aged adult population. The later years of life are marked by substantial physical changes in the body, and also by social changes as families grow away from their elderly parents, who in their turn face increasing dependency upon their adult sons and daughters. Changes such as retirement, moving home and bereavement require great adaptation on the part of the elderly. A model of nursing therefore needs to acknowledge the rapidly changing nature of an elderly person's life. It is easy to think of the elderly as static and unchanging. Once that mistake has been made, the nurse is no longer thinking of an elderly person as a living human being, rather that person has become fossilized. A developmental perspective is therefore essential that acknowledges the dynamic, changing nature of the patient's world, whatever their age.

One final area that has to be discussed is the question of how 'user friendly' the model is. Hospital wards are very busy places and theoreticians should temper their deliberations with a healthy dose of realism. This suggests that a model should be capable of providing a comprehensive assessment, but in a reasonable amount of time, and producing a care plan that is practical. Excessive use of jargon is counterproductive, although there is no reason why nurses should not convert difficult language into more readily understood English whatever the model.

For the successful use of a model, both nurse and patient need to be able to see the practical relevance of its ideas and concepts to the real world.

Summary The ideal model of nursing for adult general wards should have the following characteristics.

(1) It needs to show the patient as an integrated, individual human being with psychological and social components. Problems in these fields must be readily identified.

(2) It should permit immediate identification of physiological problems, particularly relating to life-threatening conditions involving the respiratory and cardiovascular systems, and also pain.

(3) The model must have a developmental dimension allowing for ageing and its associated changes.

(4) The ability of the patient to function outside the hospital must be a key element in care; models therefore should ideally be applicable in a community setting as well as in hospital.

(5) There needs to be emphasis on health education and patient teaching.
(6) The patient's point of view must be recognized as important and actively fed into the care planning process. Questions such as why the patient holds a point of view need to be explored.
(7) The model must be realistic and practical to apply.

The four models of nursing that are to be considered in this chapter will each be applied in turn to two different but representative patients. The reader is invited to test the models against the above list, adding ideas of their own as appropriate.

Example 1: The Orem model in acute medicine; John Harper

John Harper is a 55-year-old married bus driver with a history of angina and mild hypertension. He awoke this morning feeling unwell and collapsed with severe gripping central chest pain. His wife dialled 999 and he was brought to A&E where a medical diagnosis of acute myocardial infarction was made and he was admitted to CCU after 5 mg IV diamorphine and 12.5 mg IM prochloperazine were given. There follows an assessment and care plan based on Orem's model which could be adapted to suit many patients with an acute medical condition who are largely confined to bed.

Normal self-care ability (prior to admission)	Current self-care ability (after admission)	Self-care deficit (patient problem)
AERATION Breathing normal except on exertion when becomes short of breath (SOB) and develops chest pain which is relieved by rest and GTN. Smokes 20/day, has smokers' cough at times, no sputum at present.	RR 12, shallow. Skin pale. BP 90/60 P86 Unable to cough. ECG sinus rhythm occasional vent ectopics, ST elevation II, III, aVf. No pain at present.	(1) Inadequate ventilation (A). (2) Unstable heart rate, possible arrhythmias (P). (3) Unable to cough (A). (4) Chest pain (P).
FLUID BALANCE Normal intake of fluid except likes a few pints of beer several times a week. No probs passing urine, gets up once a night to p.u.	Too drowsy to drink, feels nauseous. Cannot walk to toilet.	(5) Unable to drink at present (A) (6) Cannot p.u. in toilet (A). (7) Feels nauseous (A).
NUTRITION Ht 5ft 8in Wt 90 kg Pays little heed to GP advice. High saturated fat low roughage diet. Bowels irregular.	Too drowsy to eat. Cannot walk to toilet.	(8) Cannot walk to toilet (A). (9) Poor diet (A,L). (10) Overweight (A,L). (11) Constipation (A,L).
ACTIVITY/REST Works as bus driver. Hobbies: plays darts for pub, watches TV a lot, supports local football team. Sleeps well, 7 hrs.	Drowsy, sleepy. Bed rest 48 hrs.	(12) Pressure sores (P). (13) Inadequate exercise (A,L).

Normal self-care ability (prior to admission)	Current self-care ability (after admission)	Self-care deficit (patient problem)
SOLITUDE/SOCIALIZATION Married, 2 married sons both live near. Outgoing popular man. Owns own house.	Not saying much as drowsy. Looks anxiously around CCU when eyes open.	(14) Feelings of isolation in unfamiliar surroundings (P).
HAZARDS Has not paid heed to GP advice re diet, smoking, drinking, etc.	Sleepy and drowsy, though appears oriented at present.	(15) May fall if tries to get out of bed (P).
NORMALCY Happy person, jokes about being overweight and BP/angina problems.	Anxious, has asked 'Am I going to die?' but said later 'Don't feel right here, let me go home.'	(16) Anxious about being in CCU/diagnosis (A).
DEVELOPMENTAL Recently became grandfather, delighted! No worries re job, bought council house had lived in for 14 years.	Realizes seriousness of condition, anxious about death.	(17) Anxious about diagnosis (A). (18) May become depressed (P,L).
HEALTH DEVIANCY Reluctant to see GP. Takes GTN for angina, Atenolol for BP. See 'Hazards'.	Occluded coronary artery for which is receiving streptokinase therapy. Diamorphine prescribed for pain IM.	(19) Bleeding disorder (P). (20) Chest pain (P). (21) Non-compliance with health education advice (P,L).

The care plan needs to take the 21 problems identified here and prioritize them. The six long-term problems are unlikely to be of much significance during his 24–28 hours on CCU, which leaves 15 short-term problems that need to be ordered in some sort of priority. The reader should consider how many of these could be included in a standardized care plan for any patient on CCU, and also how many are relevant when the patient moves to a general ward.

Care plan from 10:00 25/11/90

Problem	Goal	Nursing care
(1) Cardiac arrhythmias (P).	(a) Sinus rhythm. (b) P 70–85. BP 95/60–130/90.	1. Continual 3-lead ECG monitor. 2. Bed rest. 3. Give medication as prescribed. 4. Record P, BP hourly. 5. Give correct medication.
(2) Unable to maintain normal respiration (A).	RR 12–18.	1. Monitor RR, inform Dr if <12. 2. Give O$_2$ via nasal canulae 40%, 4L/min.
(3) Chest pain which Pt cannot relieve (P).	No pain will be felt.	1. Reduce anxiety (see (4)). 2. Give analgesia prn. 3. Ensure comfort.
(4) Anxiety (A).	Pt will state understands what is happening.	1. Give explanations about equipment and progress. 2. Encourage Pt to ask and answer, questions. 3. Keep family informed of progress, visiting times, etc.

Problem	Goal	Nursing care
(5) Bleeding due to streptokinase (P).	Pt will not suffer internal haemorrhage	1. Monitor stools for occult blood, urine for haematuria. 2. Check for headaches.
(6) Unable to maintain fluid balance (A).	Intake of 2.5L fluid/24 hrs.	1. Monitor & care for IVI. 2. Offer oral fluids (see 7:2). 3. Give anti-emetics. 4. Fluid balance chart.
(7) Feels nauseous (A).	Pt will not vomit.	1. Give anti-emetics. 2. Small sips of oral fluids.
(8) Cannot walk to toilet.	Urine output >1.5L/day.	1. Put urinal in convenient place. 2. Monitor urine output. 3. Ensure privacy while in use.
(9) Unable to relieve pressure on bony prominences.	Pt will not develop red or broken areas of skin.	1. Turn 2-hourly. 2. Encourage Pt to turn self. 3. Explain need for turning.
(10) Unable to attend to personal hygiene.	Pt will state is satisfied with hygiene.	1. Bed bath. 2. Progressively encourage Pt to wash self, etc.

The care plan outlined above sufficed for the first 24 hours on CCU. As Mr Harper had no further complications he was moved onto the open ward on his second day. At this stage the priorities in his care changed significantly, with only problems (1), (3), (4) and (5) remaining significant in his subsequent recovery phase. However, the following new problems became of importance on the ward.

Problem	Goal	Nursing care
(11) Pt anxious and withdrawn (A).	Pt will talk about why he is so anxious.	1. Discuss progress with Pt in privacy. 2. Ask if he wants to ask any questions. 3. Talk with family.
(12) Pt fears he is useless now. Afraid of sex & losing job (A).	Pt understands can continue 'normal' independent life.	1. Allow Pt to talk about worries. 2. Discuss cardiac rehab. programme. 3. Offer health ed. leaflets. 4. Involve family in discussions. 5. Introduce Pt to another who has made good recovery. 6. Emphasize positive action as in prob. (13). 7. Refer for cardiac rehab. programme.
(13) Has shown a lack of motivation to follow health education advice re smoking, diet, alcohol intake & exercise (A).	(a) Pt will discuss these topics and how they effect his condition.	1. Talk to Pt/wife, review Universal S/C demands from health ed. perspective, encourage questions. 2. Give Pt health ed. leaflets. 3. Discuss medication for angina & BP.
	(b) Pt will agree series of goals with wife to (i) stop smoking, (ii) lose 10 kg in 4 months, (iii)	1. As above. 2. Negotiate goals that are acceptable to Pt/wife, such as (i)–(iv).

Normal self-care ability (prior to admission)	Current self-care ability (after admission)	Self-care deficit (patient problem)
	reduce alcohol intake by 50%, (iv) change diet to high-fibre low-saturated fat.	3. Make appointment to see dietician. 4. Refer cardiac rehab.

Example 2: The Orem model in trauma care; Mabel Bush

Mabel Bush is an 81-year-old widow who lives alone in her own house. She fell during the night, sustaining an intertrochanteric fracture of her left femur and lay on the floor until a neighbour found her this morning. Her medical notes indicate that she has been treated for atrial fibrillation and heart failure requiring two admissions in the last 3 years, her latest being 6 months ago when she was discharged on a regime of frusemide, digoxin and potassium supplements in the form of effervescent tablets. She was admitted to the ward at 13:30 from A&E and has been scheduled for internal fixation on tomorrow morning's operating list.

Assessment at 14·00 on admission 22/8/90

Normal self-care ability (prior to admission)	Current self-care ability (after admission)	Self-care deficit (patient problem)
AERATION Breathless if has to walk more than 20 yds on flat. Only takes stairs slowly. Non-smoker. 'A bit chesty in winter'.	RR 22 sounds 'rattly', no cough, skin pale. BP 110/60, P 98 irreg. T=35.5°C.	(1) Unable to maintain adequate circulation due to heart failure. (2) Chest infection (P).
FLUID BALANCE Complains of going to toilet a lot especially at night so does not drink much in case of accidents. Has little idea of when to take frusemide.	Skin appears very dry. Immobile in traction making drinking very difficult. Clothes were wet with urine on admission, passed 80 ml of cloudy urine, protein++, offensive smell.	(3) Appears dehydrated, unable to achieve own rehydration (A). (4) Urine infection is probable (A). (5) Unable to p.u. on her own (A).
NUTRITION Ht 5ft 0in Wt 40–45 kg (estimated) looks frail. Does not bother to cook for self often. Snack diet low in roughage, vits, protein. Constipation for which takes liquid paraffin.	Not interested in food. Bowels last open 2 days ago, no urge to defecate at present.	(6) Constipation (A). (7) Poor diet leading to malnourishment (A,L).
ACTIVITY/REST Manages stairs slowly, good manual dexterity. Can only walk 20 yds with aid of stick (see aeration). Poor sleeper, catnaps during day. Reads a lot, enjoys needlework, knitting.	#L femur, pain rated 2 on a 5-point scale. Hamilton Russell traction to left leg, cannot turn in bed. Norton Score=12. Cannot wash self except hands & face.	(8) Pain which she cannot relieve (A). (9) Cannot prevent pressure sores developing (P). (10) Cannot see to personal hygiene (A).
SOLITUDE/SOCIALIZATION Lives alone. No family in area. Neighbour sees she is OK each	No family notified yet. Neighbour has locked up house, has been told	(11) Family/friends unaware she is in hospital (A).

Normal self-care ability (prior to admission)	Current self-care ability (after admission)	Self-care deficit (patient problem)
day, shops for her once/week. Sees old friends once/twice week. Admits lonely at times.	by A&E of diagnosis.	(12) May become lonely (P).
HAZARDS Worried about living alone in big house, has been afraid of falling.	Confined to bed by injury & traction. Will need surgery and general anaesthetic (GA).	(13) Risks of surgery under GA tomorrow (P).
NORMALCY Feels isolated since husband died 5 years ago, misses him a great deal. Feels the world just passes her by now.	'I want to go home'. Very tearful, does not understand or ?accept her injury despite pain.	(14) Anxious and distressed (A). (15) Lack of understanding may lead to confusion (P).
DEVELOPMENTAL Widowed 5 years, retired 21 years. Two sons, one lives Australia, other 200 miles away with own family. No close family just some old friends.	Very distressed now. 'I don't want to be a burden, I've had a long life, there's nobody left, just let me die'.	(16) Sees no point in living, lacks motivation to carry on (A).
HEALTH DEVIANCY Does not like doctors, rarely sees GP. Is not aware of effects of medication she is on or of correct time/dose.	Hamilton Russell traction for #L femur. Does not appear to accept injury. ECG=atrial fibrillation.	(17) Will not follow prescribed medication (P,L). (18) Does not accept or understand injury (A).

Care plan 14:00 22/8/90 to surgery 11:00 (approx) 23/8/90

Problem	Goal	Nursing care
(1) Pain which Pt cannot relieve (A).	Pt will be pain free.	1. Give prn analgesia as needed. 2. Apply H.R. traction L. leg. 3. Try to reduce anxiety. 4. Ensure comfort.
(2) Pt appears very distressed and anxious (A).	Pt will appear calm and talk about her fears.	1. Listen to what Pt is saying. 2. Try to see things from her point of view. 3. Offer explanations and answer questions. 4. Contact son. 5. See prob. (1).
(3) Pt unable to prevent pressure sores (P).	Skin will be unbroken, no red areas.	1. 2-hr pressure care. 2. Ripple mattress. 3. Check traction 2-hrly. 4. Sheepskin for R heel/sacrum.
(4) Pt unable to maintain hydration (A).	Fluid intake 2.5L by 11:00.	1. Explain importance of oral hydration to Pt. 2. Provide drinks she likes. 3. Encourage drinking. 4. Fluid balance chart. 5. Discuss IVI with Dr if 1–3 not successful.
(5) Urinary infection.	Pt will have no UTI in 5/7.	1. Take MSU. 2. See prob. (4). 3. Administer antibiotics.

Problem	Goal	Nursing care
(6) Unable to maintain continence (P).	No incontinence of urine.	1. Use slipper bedpan. 2. Offer to Pt hourly. 3. Give Pt nurse call buzzer. 4. Ensure privacy when on bedpan.
(7) Unable to maintain good circulation (A).	Good cardiac output as shown by P60–80, reg. BP120/60–150/90, RR<22.	1. Monitor BP, RR, P 2–4 hrly. 2. Support back with pillows in sitting position. 3. Give medication as prescribed.
(8) May lose orientation, confusion (P).	Will be oriented in time & space.	1. Give detailed explanations. 2. Ensure spectacles available. 3. Keep informed of time.
(9) Hazards of surgery under GA on 23/8/90.	Pt will have no complications from surgery.	1. NBM from 05:00. 2. IVI overnight (see prob. (4)). 3. Follow standard pre-op prep. 4. Discuss surgery with Pt.
(10) Pt unable to maintain own hygiene (A).	Will state she is satisfied with hygiene.	1. Give bed bath. 2. Encourage maximum self-care during bed bath.

The care plan above took the patient through to surgery on 23/8/90. Some problems resolved and could be dropped from the care plan, i.e. (5), (7), (8), (9) and (10). Assessment carried out on 24/8/90 after surgery revealed the following new problems which had to be added to the care plan.

Problem	Goal	Nursing care
(11) Wound over L hip.	Wound will heal by 3/9/90 with no infection.	1. Care of wound drains. 2. Remove drains if drainage <25 ml/12 hr. 3. Monitor wound dressing for signs of infection, change only if needs changing. 4. Remove sutures when Dr instructs.
(12) Pt has chest infection.	RR & T will be normal in 5/7.	1. Monitor vital signs 4-hrly. 2. Encourage coughing, deep breathing between physio visits. 3. Sit upright. 4. Give medication as prescribed.
(13) Pt reluctant to mobilize.	Pt will walk 20 yds with zimmer by 29/8/90.	1. Explain advantages of mobility. 2. Offer encouragement. 3. Ensure analgesia given 1 hr before exercise. 4. Set limited goals day by day.
(14) Pt reluctant to drink.	Fluid intake 2.5L oral/day.	1. Explain importance of drinking. 2. Ensure ready access to toilet. 3. Fluid balance chart. 4. Ensure drinks are what she likes. 5. Give frequent encouragement.
(15) Pt is eating very little.	Dietary intake of 2000C/day by 29/8/90.	1. Discuss importance of eating. 2. Offer small meals more often.

Problem	Goal	Nursing care
		3. Find out preferred foods.
		4. Provide dietary supplements in form of drinks.
		5. Consult dietitian.
(16) Pt is tearful at times and withdrawn.	Pt will talk of future plans in positive way.	1. Spend time finding out her point of view & listening to her.
		2. Encourage son to visit.
		3. Enquire if she wishes to see a minister of religion.
		4. Talk positively of the future but realistically.
		5. Contact social worker to see what support is needed/available.
		6. Encourage maximum independence while in ward.
		7. Try and give Pt sense of control over what is happening, involve in all decisions.
(17) Pt has poor knowledge of medication.	Pt will state purpose, dose & time of different drugs by discharge.	1. Tell Pt about drugs as given.
		2. On 30/8/90 give teaching session.
		3. On 31/8/90 check how much remembered.
		4. Reinforce teaching on subsequent days.
		5. Provide written instructions.

In examples 1 and 2, the Orem assessment headings have been adapted so that the four universal self-care needs of intake of air, water, food and excretion have been amended to the three headings of aeration, fluid balance and nutrition. This has been done to give a more integrated approach to each of the three basic physiological parameters of air, food and water. The concept of aeration more accurately describes what the body is actually doing, as simply taking air into the body is only the beginning of a complex process involving both the cardiovascular and respiratory systems.

Example 3:   **The Roy adaptation model in surgery; Charlie Hackworth**

Charlie Hackworth is a 74-year-old married man who has been admitted for a right below-knee amputation due to peripheral vascular disease. He has been diagnosed diabetic for 8 years, for which he takes glibenclamide and relies on diet for control. This assessment was carried out on 20/2/90 after he had been admitted for surgery the following day. As an area of maladaptive or problem behaviour is described in the first-level assessment it is underlined and numbered[1]. The second-level assessment then focuses on that behaviour and seeks to explain it in accordance with Roy's ideas of immediate cause (focal stimulus), environmental factors (contextual stimulus) and previous experiences, attitudes and beliefs (residual stimulus). As far as possible the nursing care should be designed around the second-level assessment which is attempting to discover the causes of the patient's problems. Standard pre- and post-op care plans using Roy's model can be found on p. 71.

First-level assessment	*Second-level assessment*		
	Focal	*Contextual*	*Residual*
(1) PHYSIOLOGY *Oxygenation:* RR20 <u>BP180/100 P84</u>① <u>Smoked 30/day for 60 years.</u>② Occasional cough. L foot cold, gangrenous 3–5th toes, R foot cool, pulse weak.③	(1) Cardiovascular disease.	Diabetes. Smoker.	Belief smoking does no harm.
	(2) Addiction to nicotine.		See (1).
	(3) See (1).	See (1).	See (1).
Fluid balance: Appears hydrated. Drinks average <u>12 pts beer/wk,</u>④ does not like coffee. *Nutrition:* Ht 6ft 0in Wt 92 kg	(4) Enjoys beer.	Likes pub company.	Belief drinking does no harm.
	(5) Poor diet.	Wife does all cooking.	Traditional beliefs about diet.
Looks <u>overweight,</u>⑤ admits he eats a lot of sweet food, but protests he eats little bread, only a few chips, no rice or pasta. <u>Has poor knowledge of current thinking on dietary control of diabetes.</u>⑥	(6) Has not bothered to update on current thought.	Does not like GP so reluctant to attend.	See (5).
Elimination: Bowels open every 2 days, no problems. <u>Difficulty in starting passing urine, has to get up every night, some dribbling.</u>⑦	(7) Prostatic enlargement.		
Rest & exercise: Sleeps 7 hrs a night. Can <u>only walk 50 yds</u>⑧ when calf pain forces him to stop.	(8) Intermittent claudication.		
Regulation: <u>Pain on walking</u>⑨ in L leg. Non-insulin-dependent <u>diabetes</u>⑩ since 1982. Good hearing, glasses worn for reading. <u>T 37.3°C</u>⑪.	(9) See (8). (10) Failure of pancreas to make enough insulin. (11) Infection of gangrenous toes.	Overweight	See (5)
(2) SELF-CONCEPT *Physical:* Understands will have below-knee amputation. Very <u>worried how he will manage</u>⑫ to get about, especially stairs. <u>Anxious</u>⑬ in case other leg goes the same way. Sickened by sight⑭ of L. foot.	(12) Loss of leg. (13) Fears spread of disease. (14) Gangrene	Large 3-storey house. Has seen another Pt with bilateral amputation.	Fear 'I am rotting away'.
Personal: Feels he just will not be the same person, <u>very anxious</u>⑮ will wake up in op.	(15) Fear of anaesthetic.		Heard of Pts waking up during ops.
(3) INTERDEPENDENCY Always been self-reliant, does not	(16) Hospitalization for surgery	Wife lives 20 miles away, no car.	Believes it is his job to look after her.

First-level assessment	Second-level assessment		
	Focal	*Contextual*	*Residual*

want to cause any bother to people. Feels his wife depends on him a lot, anxious⟨16⟩ how she will cope while he is in hospital.

(4) ROLE FUNCTION Retired engineer though very active still as odd job man. Father of 3 children who all live nearby, enjoys being granddad. <u>Worried how they will think of him now.</u> ⟨17⟩	(17) Surgery.		Fears he may become a burden on family.

There are three components in writing a care plan for Charlie: the need to prepare him safely for surgery tomorrow, the need to plan care that will deal with the effects of surgery, and finally the need to tackle the long-term health problems that will remain after discharge.

Pre-op care plan

Problem	Goal	Nursing care
(1) Abnormal blood sugar levels (P).	Capillary blood glucose (CBG) 4–9 mmol/L	1. Give medication. 2. Check CBG level 4-hrly. 3. Ensure correct diet. 4. Care of insulin/glucose IVI when NBM.
(2) Anxiety and fear (A).	Pt will talk of his fears.	1. Encourage Pt to talk. 2. Discuss how wife will manage without him. 3. Discuss his role in the family. 4. Talk positively about artificial leg and the advantages of increased mobility and less pain. 5. Teach about what to expect pre- and post-op. 6. Cover L. foot with dressing.
(3) Poor circulation to lower limbs (A).	R. foot still shows no signs of gangrene.	1. Avoid trauma to foot. 2. Discuss measures that can be taken by Pt after discharge to care for foot.
(5) Difficulty passing urine (P).	Pt will pass 1L urine by 08:00 . . . [tomorrow's date].	1. Encourage upright position when using bottle. 2. Show where toilets are. 3. Fluid intake >1L by 24:00.
(5) Hazards of going for surgery (P).	Pt will suffer no avoidable complications.	1. Follow standard pre-op preparation. 2. See probs. (1) & (2).

When a patient has had surgery, it is essential that there should be a thorough reassessment on return to the ward. In Charlie's case this led to the following new data being fed into his assessment sheet.

First-level assessment	Second-level assessment		
	Focal	Contextual	Residual
PHYSIOLOGY	(1) Narcotic anal-		
Oxygenation: BP135/75, P84, <u>RR12</u>①.	gesia.		
Looks pale.	(2) Post-op nausea.	Very drowsy.	
Fluid balance: <u>NBM</u>② IVI 1L/8 hr.			
Nutrition: <u>NBM.</u> ③	(3) See (2).		
Elimination: <u>Catheterized, therefore</u> <u>access for bacteria to urinary tract.</u>④	(4) To facilitate surgery.	Cross infection from other sources on ward.	
Good ouput 50–75 ml/hr.			
Rest & exercise: <u>Very drowsy</u>⑤	(5) Anaesthetic.		
<u>L below knee amputation, stump</u> <u>dressing, 2 drains.</u>⑥	(6) Surgery.	Pt is diabetic & has peripheral vascular disease.	
Regulation: Omnopon infusion for pain control, drowsy, but agrees when asked if in <u>pain</u>⑦ rated 3 on a 5-point scale.	(7) Surgery.	Pt is anxious.	
SELF CONCEPT	(8) Phantom limb.		
Physical: <u>Can still feel leg.</u>⑧			
Personal: 'Glad it's all over'.			
ROLE FUNCTION & INTERDEPENDENCE			
No change, very drowsy.			

The post-op care plan saw the following problems added onto the pre-op plan. In the first 24–48 hours problems (1) to (3) and (6) to (13) were of the greatest importance, but as his recovery progressed (6)–(13) became less relevant and problems (14)–(17) took over from them as the focus of Charlie's care. It should be noted that problems (1)–(3) were important throughout Charlie's stay in hospital.

Problem	Goal	Interventions
(6) Post-op shock (P).	BPsyst >100.	1. Maintain IVI as per chart. 2. Monitor BP, P, RR prn ½–4-hrly. 3. Observe stump bandage, wound drain for excess bleeding.
(7) Respiratory depression (P).	RR>10.	1. See (6)2. 2. Give O_2 as prescribed.
(8) Pain (A).	Pt will state is pain free.	1. Monitor pain levels ½-hrly. 2. Give analgesia as required. 3. Give information, reduce anxiety.
(9) Dehydration (P).	Fluid intake >2.5L/day.	1. Care of IVI. 2. Fluid balance chart. 3. Encourage oral fluids.
(10) Failure of wound to heal properly (P).	Would will heal without infection in 14 days.	1. Monitor wound drains. 2. Remove if drainage <25 ml/ 12 hr. 3. Leave dressing untouched as long as possible.

Problem	Goal	Interventions
		4. Change bandage prn.
		5. Monitor temp. 4-hrly.
		6. Remove sutures in accordance with surgeon's instructions.
(11) Chest infection (P).	No chest infection.	1. Encourage deep breathing coughing exercises.
		2. Nurse in upright position.
		3. Encourage mobility, see (12).
(12) Immobility (A).	No pressure sores, DVT/PE, hip contractures will occur.	1. Turn 2-hrly.
		2. Explain need for Pt to move self around in bed.
		3. Sit out of bed 1 hr 1st day post-op.
		4. Lie face down twice daily ½ hr
		5. Carefully apply TED stocking to R. Leg.
		6. Monitor pressure areas 2-hrly.
		7. Use wheelchair when able.
		8. Discuss temporary prosthesis.
(13) Urinary tract infection (P).	No urine infection will occur.	1. Catheter care prn.
		2. Fluid intake >2.5L/day after catheter removed.
(14) Smokes 30/day (AL).	Will give up.	1. Discuss & provide health ed. literature.
(15) Overweight (AL).	Will lose 10 kg from post-op wt in 4 wks.	1. Teach about diet.
		2. Arrange for dietitian to see Pt and wife together.
		3. Order correct diet.
		4. See (17).
(16) Poor dietary control of diabetes (AL).	Will describe correct diet by discharge.	1. See (15).
(17) Drinks too much alcohol — 25 units/wk (AL).	Will reduce intake by 50% to 12 units per week after discharge.	1. Health ed. advice.
		2. Discuss low-alcohol beers.

Example 4: Roy's adaptation model in surgery; Margaret Hill

Margaret Hill is a 58-year-old woman who has been diagnosed as having cancer of the rectum. She has been admitted for anterior resection of the rectum and temporary formation of a colostomy. In the previous example we saw how the care plan was built of two components, pre-op and post-op, based on two separate assessments; the same approach will be used here. The following assessment was therefore carried out on admission the day before surgery.

First-level assessment	Second-level assessment		
	Focal	*Contextual*	*Residual*
PHYSIOLOGICAL *Oxygenation*: RR16 <u>BP165/70 P94;</u>① non-smoker, warm dry skin. *Fluid balance*: Looks well hydrated, occasional alcohol. *Nutrition*: Ht 5ft 5in Wt 50 kg. Has <u>lost weight recently.</u>② Poor diet low in roughage.③ *Elimination*: No problems with passing urine. Seems <u>embarrassed</u>④ to talk of bowels. Last 6/12 <u>constipation and diarrhoea</u>⑤ with some blood staining. Has <u>always had a tendency to be constipated.</u>⑥ *Rest & exercise*: <u>Sleeps poorly</u>⑦ since death of husband. Fully mobile, enjoys reading, TV, knitting. *Regulation*: Had hysterectomy 9 years ago. T=36.8°C. Wears glasses for read- ing.	(1) Anxiety and fear. (2) Lost appetite. (3) Lack of know- ledge. (4) Belief it is not polite. (5) Cancer of rectum. (6) Lack of know- ledge about diet. (7) Death of husband	Ward environment. Suffering from cancer, see (3). Lack of motivation since husband died last year.	Had hysterectomy 9 years ago, very painful. Fears death. Traditional beliefs re diet.
SELF CONCEPT *Physical*: Feels she got over her hyster- ectomy, relieved it stopped her menstrual problems. <u>Very worried about stoma</u>⑧ formation, 'But if it has to be done, it has to be done'. *Personal*: <u>Afraid cancer will kill her,</u>⑨ worried it has spread already, also afraid it might return elsewhere. A neighbour died in this way. **ROLE FUNCTION**: Widowed 12 months. Has 3 married children who live in the area, close supportive family. Works as part time shop assistant. <u>Admits to feeling</u>⑩ <u>lost without her husband,</u> lets things drift along, still cries over him, visits his grave and 'talks to him'. She became very tearful at this point. **INTERDEPENDENCE**: Tries to be independ- ent. 'I don't want to bother anybody'. Acknowledges children have own lives to live. This was said with some sadness as if she finds it <u>hard to adapt</u>⑪ to children's independence.	(8) Probable stoma formation after resection of rectum. (9) Cancer. (10) Grieving for husband. (11) Children have become in- dependent of her.	Afraid people will smell it.	Embarrassed about bowel function. Experience of seeing a neighbour die of cancer. Needs to feel wanted as a mother, especially since widowed.

This assessment led to the following pre-op care plan being written.

Problem	Goal	Nursing care
(1) Anxiety due to fear of: (a) surgery, (b) cancer, (c) effects of stoma, (d) further erosion of her role in the family (A).	(a) Pt will talk of her fears pre- & post-op. (b) Pt will appear positive in talking of these problems by discharge.	1. Give information. 2. Encourage questions. 3. Stoma specialist to see Pt pre-op. 4. Discuss (a)–(d) with sensitivity and in private.
(2) Complications of surgery (P).	Pt will suffer no avoidable problems.	1. Standard pre-op procedure.
(3) Pt may develop peritonitis due to contamination of surgical field by faeces.	Rectum and bowel will be empty of faeces.	1. Bowel washout today x2 and in morning. 2. Fluids only.

Mrs Hill was then reassessed on return from theatre the following day after resection of her rectum and stoma formation.

First-level assessment	Focal	Contextual	Residual
		Second-level assessment	
PHYSIOLOGICAL *Oxygenation:* BP95/60 P98 RR18.① Breathing shallow.②	(1) Hypovolaemia. (2) Pain.	Moderate pain. Post G.A.	
Fluids: NBM③ Blood transfusion running.	(3) No bowel sounds.	Nauseated.	
Nutrition: NBM④	(4) See (3).		
Elimination: Urinary catheter good output. Naso-gastric tube mod drainage. Colostomy L. lower quadrant.⑤ Looks pink, bag empty. Two wound drains from lower abdominal wound, slight oozing.⑥	(5) Surgery for cancer. (6) See (5).		
Rest & activity: Drowsy, reluctant to move in bed.⑦	(7) Pain.	Afraid of 'drips and drains'.	
Regulation: Pain⑧ is rated 3 on a 5-point scale. T 36.9°C.	(8) Surgery.	Anxiety.	Frightened to ask for analgesia.
SELF CONCEPT *Physical:* Has refused to look at stoma.⑨	(9) Embarrassed.	Already very stressed 'I've been through enough today'.	
Personal: Relieved it is all over.			
INTERDEPENDENCE Has not asked for help despite pain.⑩	(10) Desire to maintain independence.		
ROLE FUNCTION Family anxious to see her.			

Margaret's care plan was therefore added to, reflecting immediate post-op priorities (problems (4)–(10)) but with long-term problems such as (1), (9) and (11) figuring increasingly in care as she recovers from the immediate effects of surgery.

Problem	Goal	Nursing care
(4) Pain (A).	Pt will state she has no pain.	1. Monitor pain levels with 5-point scale. 2. Give analgesia as needed. 3. Give information and try to reduce anxiety. 4. Make comfortable. 5. Discuss importance of asking for analgesia.
(5) Hypovolaemic shock (P).	BPsyst>90.	1. Ensure IVI runs to time. 2. Record BP, P, RR ½-hrly. 3. Monitor wound & drains.
(6) Dehydration (P).	Fluid intake >2.5L/day.	1. Fluid balance chart.
(7) Nausea and vomiting (A).	Pt will not vomit.	1. Nasogastric tube free drainage. 2. NBM until bowel sounds return. 3. Give anti-emetics prn.
(8) Pt is not able to eat.	Will start light diet within 4 days.	1. Keep hydrated, See (6). 2. Ask what she likes. 3. Discuss diet and stoma. 4. Avoid nausea, see (7). 5. Offer supplement drinks.
(9) Failure of colostomy to work (P).	Stoma will start to work <3 days.	1. Check appearance of stoma is normal. 2. Ask Pt if she feels any wind. 3. Listen for bowel sounds.
(10) Pt is unable to accept stoma (A).	(a) Pt wil look at stoma <3 days. (b) Pt will help nurse change bag <6 days. (c) Pt will change bag alone before discharge.	1. Encourage and discuss stoma with Pt. 2. Make it an ordinary part of care, i.e. no gloves, normal facial expression. 3. Stoma specialist to visit. 4. Arrange visit from other stoma patient. 5. Talk to family about stoma at visiting times. 6. Reinforce temporary nature of colostomy.
(11) Surgical wound (A).	Would will heal without complications 14 days.	1. Remove wound drains when drainage <25 ml in 12 hrs. 2. Do not disturb dressing unless necessary. 3. Monitor T 4-hrly if >37°C. 4. Remove sutures according to surgeon's instructions.
(12) Pt lacks motivation and has tended to neglect self since being widowed.	Pt will express positive views about going home.	1. Allow her to talk of her husband. 2. Discuss her job with her. 3. Reinforce temporary nature of stoma. 4. Encourage visiting by family. 5. Explore new things she could do with her life, new interests.

Mrs Hill also had problems surrounding her inability to maintain personal hygiene and potential problems of chest infection, pressure sores, DVT, and urinary tract infection from an indwelling catheter. Reference is made to the previous care plan (Charlie Hackworth) to see how these may be dealt with.

Standard pre-op care plan based on Roy's adaptation model

N.B. As a standardized care plan all the problems are potential. Such a care plan should be completed with individualized problems specific to each patient.

Problem	Adaptation Goal	Intervention
PHYSIOLOGICAL MODE		
(1) *Respiratory.*		
(a) Asphyxia due to blockage of airway by vomitus, saliva or false teeth while Pt unconscious.	Airway will remain patent.	1. NBM 4-hr pre-op. 2. Remove and label dentures pre-op. 3. Note capped teeth.
(b) Post-op chest infection due to:	No post-op chest inf.	
(i) Smoking		1. Discuss post-op risks of continuing. 2. Negotiate reduction or cessation if sufficient time pre-op.
(ii) Poor lung expansion		1. Teach deep breathing & coughing exercises, explain importance. 2. Refer physio. encourage exercises. 3. Baseline RR obs.
(iii) Pre-op upper resp. tract infection.		1. Baseline T, P, RR. 2. Observe for signs of cough or shortness of breath.
(2) *Circulatory*		
(a) Cardiovascular complications under GA.	No complications will occur under GA.	1. Baseline P, BP obs. 2. Check 12 lead ECG carried out.
(b) DVT/PE post-op due to immobility.	No DVT or PE will develop.	1. Discuss risks with Pt. 2. Teach and practise leg exercise. 3. Teach about TED stockings.
(3) *Fluids* Dehydration if NBM >6 hrs (see (1)a).	24 hr pre-op intake of 2.5L.	1. Inform medical staff if Pt NBM >8 hrs. 2. Assist siting IVI. 3. Fluid balance chart.
(4) *Nutrition* See (1) a		
(5) *Elimination*		
(a) Incontinence of urine during surgery.	Pt will not be incontinent during surgery.	1. Ensure Pt voids bladder pre-op. 2. Explain about catheters if Pt likely to have catheter post-op.

Problem	Adaptation Goal	Intervention
(b) Incontinence of faeces during surgery.	Will not be incontinent during surgery.	1. Ask Pt to have bowels open pre-op. 2. Give aperient, suppositories enema prn.
(6) *Rest and activity* (a) Insomnia due to anxiety about op.	Pt will have usual amount of sleep.	1. Give Pt chance to discuss anxieties. 2. Teach about pre- and post-op care so Pt knows what to expect. 3. Give night sedation.
(b) Incorrect surgery may be performed due to mis-identification of unconscious Pt.	Pt will have correct surgery.	1. Check wrist band, notes, X-rays & consent form before Pt leaves wd.
(c) Wound infection due to contaminated skin.	No post-op wound infection.	1. Remove hair from site of surgery with depilatory cream. 2. Bath or shower, theatre gown. 3. Remove jewellery etc.
(7) *Regulation* (a) Risk of complications if Pt is undiagnosed diabetic.	No complications will occur.	1. Test urine pre-op.
(b) Errors in drug dosage due to incorrect wt.	No errors due to incorrect wt will occur.	1. Weigh Pt accurately pre-op.
(c) Pt will be anxious about post-op pain.	Pt will state s/he is less anxious.	1. Discuss post-op care and methods of pain relief with Pt. 2. Discuss pain assessment, pain ruler.
SELF-CONCEPT MODE (8) *Physical* Pt anxious re changes in body image after surgery.	Pt able describe changes that may occur.	1. Encourage Pt to talk about how see self now and after changes. 2. Describe changes. 3. Discuss coping strategies.
(9) *Personal* (a) Loss of self-esteem due to loss of privacy & independence.	Pt states is satisfied with privacy and the way they are cared for.	1. Ensure maximum privacy. 2. Consult Pt at all times in carrying out care.
(b) Fear and anxiety about surgery.	Pt shows understanding of surgery.	1. Discuss surgery with Pt and family. 2. Encourage questions, give info.
ROLE MASTERY MODE (10) Loss of control over life due to hospitalization.	Pt will feel they are in control of their life.	1. Involve Pt fully in care, encourage Pt to take responsibility.
INTERDEPENDENCE MODE (11) Anxiety concerning family while Pt is in hospital.	Pt will state they feel less anxious about family while in hospital.	1. Discuss family with Pt and how they will cope. 2. Encourage visiting.

The care plan offered here is only a suggestion, wards may add or subtract other aspects of care as they see fit.

Standard post-op care plan based on Roy's adaptation model The care plan given here is not offered as a definitive post-op standard care plan, but rather a guide to what such a plan may look like. Differing hospitals and wards will have varying approaches depending upon local circumstances.

Problem	Goal	Intervention
PHYSIOLOGICAL MODE		
(1) *Respiratory*		
(a) Blocked airway due to obstruction by tongue, vomit or secretions while Pt unconscious.	Airway will remain patent.	1. Leave Guerdal airway until Pt expels it. 2. Nurse Pt in semi-prone position. 3. Keep neck extended if Guerdal in situ. 4. Ensure suction available. 5. Remain with Pt until gag reflex has returned (NB. Above applies usually to recovery room rather than ward).
(b) Respiratory depression due to anaesthetic or narcotic drugs.	RR>12 with good tissue perfusion.	1. Monitor RR and depth. 2. Give O_2 prn.
(c) Chest infection due to retention of secretions and atelectasis.	No chest infection.	1. Encourage breathing exercises 2-hrly. 2. Nurse Pt in upright position in bed. 3. Give analgesia to assist pain-free coughing. 4. Turn Pt 2-hrly. 5. 4-hrly temp for 24 hrs. 6. Sit out of bed first post-op day.
(2) *Circulatory*		
(a) Risk of shock.	Systolic BP will remain >90.	1. Monitor P/BP/RR, skin condition ¼–½–1–2–4 hr/prn. Notify Dr if BP<90. 2. Observe dressings & wound drains for signs of excessive bleeding. 3. Monitor hrly urine output. Notify Dr if <30 ml/hr.
(b) Presence of shock.	Systolic BP will recover >90.	1. Elevate foot of bed. 2. Give high concentration O_2. 3. See prob (2). 4. IVI as per instructions.
(c) DVT due to immobility.	DVT will not occur.	1. 2-hr leg exercises. 2. TED stockings. 3. Reinforce pre-op teaching. 4. Monitor calf pain.
(d) PE 2° to a DVT.	PE will not occur.	1. See prob. (2)c.
(e) Wound may become infected.	Wound will heal without complications within 14 days.	1. Transparent dressing. 2. Change dressing only when needed. 3. Inspect for signs of infection prn. 4. 4-hr temp obs for 3 days. 5. Empty wound drains prn. 6. Remove drains when drainage ceased.

Problem	Goal	Intervention
		7. Aseptic technique at all times. 8. Remove sutures when surgeon orders.
(3) *Fluids* (a) Dehydration due to vomiting or Pt being NBM.	Fluid intake >2.5L/day.	1. Fluid balance chart. 2. Care of IVI. 3. Encourage oral fluids as per Dr's orders as bowel sounds return.
(b) Vomiting due to post-op ileus or drug side effects.	Pt will not vomit.	1. NBM. 2. Nasogastric tube on free drainage. 3. See Problem (3)a. 4. Give anti-emetics prn.
(c) Oral infection due to NBM.	Pt will not develop oral infection.	1. 4-hrly mouth toilet while NBM. 2. Ice to suck.
(4) *Nutrition* See (3)b.		
(5) *Elimination* (a) Retention of urine.	Pt will pass urine <12 hrs after theatre.	1. Assist Pt to use bottle, commode. 2. Ensure Pt knows how to ask for help. 3. Fluid balance chart.
(b) Constipation due to effects of drugs or post-op ileus.	Pt will have bowels open within 3 days of surgery.	1. Assist Pt to use commode or toilet. 2. See (3)a. 3. Consider suppositories if no bowel action at 3 days.
(6) *Rest & Activity* (a) Pt unable to maintain personal hygiene due to surgery.	Pt will state satisfied with personal hygiene.	1. Bedbath first day post-op. 2. Assist with hygiene on subsequent days encouraging maximum Pt activity. 3. Sit out in bathroom by day 4.
(b) Risk of pressure sores.	No pressure sores.	1. 2-hrly turns. 2. Encourage mobility, reinforce pre-op teaching. 3. Use of special aids if needed.
(7) *Regulation* (a) Pain due to surgery.	Pt will state pain free.	1. Give analgesia prn. 2. Offer information & psychological support. 3. Ensure Pt comfort at all times.
(b) Pyrexia due to infection.	Pt temp <37°C.	1. 4-hr temp obs. 2. If T>38°C fan therapy. 3. If T>39°C tepid sponge.
SELF-CONCEPT (8) *Physical* Distress at altered body image.	Pt will show signs of adaptation by being able to look at site of surgery and talk positively about self after surgery.	1. Reinforce pre-op teaching. 2. Encourage Pt/family to talk about surgery. 3. Invite Pt to look at wound. 4. Introduce to others with similar surgery if possible. 5. Involve family in discussion according to Pt's wishes.

Problem	Goal	Intervention

(9) *Personal*
  (a) Loss of self-esteem.
  (b) Anxiety over outcome of surgery.
	See pre-op care plan.
	
	Pt will show understanding of results of surgery.
		
		1. Discuss surgery with Pt and family. Answer questions honestly but check what info Drs have given.

ROLE FUNCTION MODEL (10) Loss of control over life.	See pre-op care plan.	
INTERDEPENDENCE MODEL (11) (a) Anxiety re family while in hospital (b) Reluctance to ask for help.	See pre-op care plan. Pt will ask for help when needed.	 1. Ensure call bell within reach. 2. Encourage Pt to ask for help.

Example 5: **The FANCAP Assessment Scheme in A&E**

Assessment in A&E is based on the well known 'ABC of resuscitation' protocol which requires airway, breathing, circulation, cervical spine and consciousness to be the first priorities. This is a tried and tested method for assessing immediate life-threatening problems; however, it does not go beyond the urgent problems. FANCAP can be used to give the same priorities as the ABC scheme, but has the advantage of exploring other areas. If the assessment begins with 'Aeration', airway, breathing and circulation will be covered; 'Activity' should make the nurse look for any signs of limb weakness or neck injury, while 'Communication' requires an assessment of level of consciousness. Pain should be assessed next, leaving fluids and nutrition until last. Thus, in A&E the FANCAP scheme becomes AACPFN, suggestions are invited for an easy way out of remembering this acronym!

Nurses in A&E rarely have the luxury of time in which to write detailed care plans and care planning is frequently done in the nurse's head rather than on paper. Standardized care plans offer one solution to this problem, even if only as teaching tools for staff new to the department or as a way of setting standards for care. Consider the following two examples which show how FANCAP may be used for two very different A&E patients.

5a. Patrick Dunne Patrick was brought to the A&E department after being found unconscious in a street, he appears rather dishevelled.

AERATION
Airway. Patent.
Breathing: RR 12 deep & regular, smells strongly of alcohol.
Circulation: BP 110/70, P 70. *Skin:* Very dirty.
Other Comments: Not expressing any emotions, uncommunicative.

ACTIVITY
Neck: No evidence of injury. *Limbs:* No voluntary movement, unresponsive, no history of trauma available, no sign of injury to limbs.
COMMUNICATION
Level of consciousness: Best response; flexes to painful stimulus, nil verbally, pupils = react briskly (see head injury chart).
Wounds: Small laceration over R eye.
Understanding of situation: Nil, unresponsive.
Eyesight: Not wearing glasses.
Hearing: Unresponsive to verbal stimulus.
PAIN
Location: Nil.
Severity 0–5: 0, unresponsive.
Type: —
Other comments: —
Anxiety: —
FLUIDS
In: Has almost empty bottle of wine in pocket.
Out: Has been incontinent of urine.
Family/friends: Nobody with him, looks to be sleeping rough.
NUTRITION
In: Appears underfed, CBG 3 mmol/L.
Out: Trousers show evidence of previous faecal incontinence, shirt soaked in fresh vomit.

This assessment should allow the nurse to deduce that Patrick's major problem is a potential threat to his airway from vomiting whilst unconscious and lead to him being positioned on his side, under observation, while he sleeps off his excess alcohol intake.

5b. Darren Mardon   This 18-year-old motorcyclist was brought to A&E after an RTA.

AERATION
Airway: Tolerates Guerdal oral airway.
Breathing: RR 30 shallow, paradoxical resps. R side of chest.
Circulation: BP 80/40, P 128. *Skin*: Pale, cold, sweaty.
Other comments: Expressing nothing verbally.
ACTIVITY
Neck: No evidence of injury but marks on crash helmet indicate substantial blow to head.
Limbs: No voluntary movement, clinically #R shaft femur, closed.
COMMUNICATION
Level of consciousness: Unresponsive to painful stimulus (see head injury chart). R pupil sluggish to react and dilated.
Wounds: Nil.
Understanding: Nil.
Eyesight: No glasses.
Hearing: Unresponsive.
PAIN
Location: Unresponsive.
Severity 0–5: 0
Type: —
Other comments: —
Anxiety: —
FLUIDS
In: Not known when last had drink.
Out: Bladder non-palpable.
Family/friends: Police are notifying his parents.
NUTRITION
In: Looks within normal range ht/wt ratio. Last ate ? when.
Out: —

This rapid assessment allowed A&E staff to identify a serious head injury, flail segment and fracture of the right femur as his main injuries. His main problems in A&E could be listed as follows:

(1) Airway obstruction (P)
(2) Hypovolaemic shock (A)
(3) Respiratory failure (A)
(4) Unconsciousness (A)
(5) Cervical spine injury (P)
(6) Fractured right femur (A)
(7) Neurovascular complications of that fracture (P)

Such an assessment revealed the urgent problems needing nursing care while resuscitation was carried out and medical diagnosis of his injuries was finalized.

It is worthwhile looking at how this scheme may now be applied to Darren's care on ITU where ventilatory support was needed due to his head and chest injuries. A Steinmann pin had been inserted in his R. tibia and sliding traction applied to stabilize his fractured R. femur. The flexibility of FANCAP is shown by this different approach to its usage on ITU.

Example 6:   Assessment of Darren Mardon on ITU

AERATION

In	*Out*
Intubated with size 9 Portex ET tube. Ventilated on preset inspired minute vol of 8L/min, RR12 Airway pressures 22–24 mmHg. 50% humidified oxygen. Both sides of chest rising equally.	BP 120/80 P86 CVP +4 (18:00hrs). ECG sinus rhythm. Two chest drains in situ. Arterial line in situ for BP.

COMMUNICATION

In	*Out*
Does not respond to verbal or painful stimulus, R. pupil remains sluggish and dilated. According to parents has no hearing or eyesight problems.	No attempt at communication with staff, unresponsive. No wounds noted.

FLUIDS

In	*Out*
NBM, Peripheral and central lines in situ. See fluid balance chart. *Social:* Family and girlfriend keen to visit	Catheter draining well 60–90 ml per hr clear urine.

PAIN

In	*Out*
Pt has suffered #R.femur. *Psychological:* No facial evidence of anxiety/fear.	Showing no visible evidence of pain, unresponsive.

ACTIVITY

In	*Out*
CBG 7.5. *Recreational:* Keen footballer. *Work:* Apprentice electrician at B&E Ltd. Works know of situation.	No voluntary movement of limbs.

NUTRITION

In	*Out*
NBM. Bowel sounds present.	Bowels not yet opened.

Problem	Goal	Intervention
(1) Airway obstruction (P).	Pt will have a patent airway.	1. Check ET tube+ connections secure. 2. ET suction hrly/prn.
(2) Pt unable to maintain adequate respiration (A).	Arterial blood gases (ABGs) within normal limits.	1. Hrly physio. 2. Monitor chest movements. 3. Monitor and adjust O_2 conc. & ventilator settings according to Dr's instructions and ABGs. 4. Give sedation as per drug chart. 5. See probs. (1)+(3).
(3) Pt may go into resp. failure due to pneumothorax (P).	No haemo/pneumothorax will recur.	1. Record chest drainage hrly. 2. Ensure drains are patent. 3. Minimal clamping of drains. 4. See prob. (2).
(4) Shock (P).	BPsyst 100–140.	1. Continuous BP monitoring. 2. Give IVI as per chart.
(5) Raised intracranial pressure (ICP) (P).	No signs of raised ICP.	1. Continuous BP monitoring. 2. Pupil obs ½-hrly.
(6) Dehydration (P).	Fluid intake 2.5L/day.	1. Give IVI as per chart. 2. Record urine output hrly. 3. CVP readings hrly. 4. Fluid balance chart.
(7) #R.Femur (A).	# will remain immobilized in correct position.	1. Check weights clear of floor. 2. Correct external rotation with padding. 3. Ensure pulley system runs free. 4. Dress pin sites as required.
(8) Neurovascular damage R.leg (P).	Good pedal pulse R.foot.	1. Care of traction as per (7). 2. Check pulse, skin colour warmth ½–4-hrly.
(9) Pain (P).	No painful expression on face.	1. Give sufficient analgesia/sedation to ensure easily ventilated & shows no pain.
(10) Pressure sores (P).	No breaks in skin will occur.	1. Pressure area care 2-hrly. 2. Ripple mattress.
(11) Stress of ITU environment (A).	Pt will suffer minimum stress and not develop stress ulceration.	1. Talk to Pt at all times as though he can hear, explaining where he is and what is happening. 2. Give ranitidine as per chart. 3. Ensure adequate periods of rest. 4. Ensure adequate sedation given. 5. Encourage visits from family & girlfriend.
(12) Unable to see to personal hygiene (A).	Will appear clean and well-groomed.	1. Bed bath daily. 2. Mouth & eye care 2-hrly.

This care plan is the broad outline of care required for Darren. The fine detail will be provided by experienced ITU staff without the need to write it down, e.g. the 'bag and suck' regime required to prevent the build up of secretions in the bronchial tree and ET tube. This may be thought of as an example of the 'expert nurse' discussed on p. 16. A care plan for an ITU patient needs to be flexible as the patient's condition may change from hour to hour and medical staff may order changes in various regimes, e.g. ventilator settings, IVIs, at the same rate or even more frequently if required. The nurse may feel there is a sufficient common core of care to make the development of standard care plans worthwhile on ITU. If so, a strong individualized component must remain.

A great deal of information is recorded at ½-hourly or hourly intervals, so accurate charting is an essential part of the assessment–care–evaluation feedback system. This also helps to explain the brief nature of the assessment given here: many of the data are already recorded on charts, there is no point in duplication. The 'In/Out' approach to assessment was more rigorously adhered to here than in the A&E examples as this concept of homeostasis is of fundamental importance in life support.

Example 7: **Roper's model on a care of the elderly unit; Jenny Haynes**

Jenny Haynes is a 78-year-old woman who was admitted after collapsing at home with a cerebrovascular accident. She has had a history of transient ischaemic attacks and has been treated for hypertension before today's episode. She also suffers from osteo-arthritis. Her daughter accompanied her to hospital and helped with the assessment.

A.L.	Usual independent routines	Problem
Maintaining a safe environment	Cares for herself at home.	May fall out of bed (P).
Communicating	Slightly deaf, has 2 pairs of glasses for short & long sight. Speech slurred at present, though understandable, due to CVA. Conscious though drowsy, appears aware of surroundings.	Slurred speech (A). Confusion (P).
Breathing	RR14 BP180/100. Non-smoker. Has history of bad colds in winter.	
Eating and drinking	Ht 5ft 0in approx, appears very overweight. 'Likes her food, always been a big eater'. Diet is low in fibre. Has not been drinking much in the evening (see elimination). Wears dentures.	Overweight (A). Dehydration (P). Poor nutrition (A).
Elimination	Sometimes has accidents with passing urine if she cannot get to toilet in time, so tends not to drink a lot in the evening. Prone to constipation.	Incontinence of urine (P). Constipation (A).

A.L.	Usual independent routines	Problem
Personal cleansing/dressing	Able to attend to own hygiene though arthritis makes it hard to bend over and reach feet.	Is unable to attend to own hygiene at present (A).
Body temperature	T 35.9°C. 'I do feel the cold in winter, it's cold now'.	Pt is cold (A).
Mobilizing	Walks slowly with aid of stick. Can manage to reach local shops which are only 50 yards away but arthritis is painful.	Has mild L hemiplegia since CVA (A). Pressure sores (P). (Norton Scale 11)
Working and playing	Watches TV and reads, used to do needlework, but hands too clumsy and painful now. OAP. Retired.	
Expressing sexuality	Still takes pride in her appearance, widowed 8 years ago. Lives with younger sister age 74.	
Sleeping	Poor sleeper.	May not sleep well (P).
Dying	Takes each day as it comes: 'At my age you know you can't go on for ever'.	

The following plan of care was devised for Mrs Haynes.

Problem	Goal	Nursing care
(1) May fall out of bed (P).	Will not fall out of bed.	1. Orientate Pt in space. 2. Cot sides at night.
(2) Slurred speech (A).	Pt will be able to make self understood.	1. Listen carefully to Pt. 2. Ask to speak slowly. 3. Explain side-effects of CVA.
(3) Confusion (P).	Pt will be oriented in time and space.	1. Reality orientation programme.
(4) Dehydration (A).	Fluid intake 3L/day.	1. Care of IVI. 2. Encourage oral fluids. 3. Fluid balance chart. 4. Explain need for oral fluids.
(5) Overweight (A).	Pt to lose 10 kg in 3 months.	1. Contact dietitian. 2. Assist with feeding. 3. Discuss healthy eating when her condition has improved.
(6) Incontinent of urine (P).	Pt will not be incontinent.	1. Give Pt call bell and explain its use; check she understands. 2. Offer bedpans 2-hrly. 3. Fluid balance chart.
(7) Constipation (A).	Pt will have bowels open within 48 hrs.	1. Ensure hydration, see (4). 2. See (5). 3. Give suppositories if no action in 48 hrs.

Problem	Goal	Intervention
(8) Unable to see to own hygiene (A).	Pt will state is satisfied with personal hygiene.	1. Bed bath including mouth and eye care. 2. Encourage maximum participation by Pt.
(9) Pt feels cold (A).	Pt will state she is not cold.	1. Supply extra bedding. 2. Check temp 4-hrly.
(10) Mild L. hemiplegia (A).	Pt will not have contractures or injury to L.limbs.	1. Discuss exercise regime with physios and carry out according to plan. 2. Approach from R. side. 3. Place cups etc. R. side.
(11) Pressure sores (P).	Pt will not develop broken skin.	1. 2-hrly pressure care. 2. Check condition of skin 2-hrly. 3. Encourage Pt mobility and explain why.
(12) Lack of sleep (A).	Pt will state she had good night's sleep.	1. Ensure quiet environment. 2. Explain what is happening at night. 3. Give medication as per chart.

One final care plan using the Roper model will be looked at before discussing the merits of these four approaches, particularly with reference to the criteria outlined on p. 53 for a good hospital model of nursing.

Example 8: **The Roper model in medical nursing; William Slater**
Bill Slater is a 68-year-old retired publican who has been admitted with acute shortness of breath and heart failure. He has had several admissions to hospital in the last few years and has a medical diagnosis of chronic obstructive airways disease (COAD) and congestive heart failure. He responded well to nebulized salbutamol therapy on admission and his breathing is now easier. This assessment was carried out a few hours after admission.

A.L.	Usual routines	Problems
Maintaining a safe environment	Lives in bungalow with wife, uncertain about his medication. Admits enjoying a few drinks, evasive as to how many. Old bruises noted on arm and face 'Fell over in the dark'.	May not understand medication correctly (P). ? Alcohol abuse (P).
Communicating	Speech laboured, SOB. Hearing good, wears reading glasses, trying to make jokes.	
Breathing	RR 24, BP 150/90. Nicotine stains on fingers, admits smokes 10–15/day. Was using accessory muscles on admission tho' breathing now easier, sounds rattly, has coughed up some green sputum.	Chest infection (A). Episodes of respiratory distress (P). Smokes (A).
Eating and drinking	Overweight, Ht 5ft 7in, weight 88 kg. Diet is high in saturated fats and refined carbohydrates, low in fruit. Drinking, see safe environment.	Overweight (A). Low-fibre diet (A).
Eliminating	No problems passing urine or faeces.	
Personal cleansing	Has bath every day, no problems.	

Problems	Goals	Nursing Care
Body temperature	Feels hot, skin is sweaty. T37.7°C axilla.	Pyrexial (A).
Mobilizing	Gets SOB after walking 100–200 yards on the flat, manages stairs slowly.	Cannot walk more than few feet at present (A).
Working and playing	Had been publican for 30 years before retired 18 months ago. Never had time for hobbies, so does little now except watch TV and read papers. Admits to being bored.	Boredom (A).
Sexuality	Sex life 'None of your business'.	
Sleeping	Used to late nights, now finds it hard to sleep, Takes tablets.	Insomnia (A).
Dying	'Never thought about it'.	

The following care plan was drawn up based on this assessment.

Problems	Goals	Nursing Care
(1) Lack of understanding of medication (A).	Pt will explain medication, dose & side-effects.	1. Discuss with Pt when he is better. 2. Give written information.
(2) Possible alcohol abuse (A).	Pt will recognize he may have a problem.	1. Observe for signs of abstinence syndrome. 2. No alcohol allowed. 3. Discuss alcohol intake at later stage when better.
(3) Chest infection (A).	Chest infection will resolve in 5 days, clear sputum.	1. Antibiotics as per chart. 2. Sit upright. 3. Encourage deep breathing & coughing. 4. Monitor RR, T 4-hrly.
(4) Respiratory distress (P).	RR<20.	1. See (3). 2. Medication as per chart. 3. See (8). 4. No smoking at present. 5. Monitor BP, P, RR 4-hrly.
(5) Smokes (A).	Pt will give up.	1. Discuss effects of smoking, give leaflets.
(6) Overweight (A).	Pt will lose 7 kg in 10 weeks.	1. Consult dietitian. 2. Discuss healthy eating.
(7) Pyrexial (A).	T<37.2°C in 5 days.	1. See (3).
(8) Limited mobility (A).	Pt will not get SOB on exertion.	1. Use commode for first 24 hrs. 2. Bed rest 24 hrs. 3. Assisted wash at bedside. 4. Allow to bathroom in 48 hrs. 5. Walk to day room in 48 hrs.
(9) Boredom.	Pt will appear to take an interest in ward activity.	1. Ensure has newspapers/books. 2. Encourage other Pts to talk to him if he is able. 3. Find time to talk to him.
(10) Insomnia.	Pt will say has slept >6 hours.	1. Ask if anything helps him sleep. 2. Minimize night noise. 3. Medication as per chart.

Discussion   It remains to conclude this chapter by seeing how the four models used compare with each other and with the criteria set on p. 53 for an ideal model of nursing in a general hospital setting.

The Orem and Roy models allowed the nurses to readily assess the key physiological aspects of the patient as did the FANCAP scheme. Flexibility in the order of assessment is essential together with a sense of priority, i.e. the most urgent things are assessed first and nurses should not be afraid to vary the order in which an assessment is carried out according to the patient's needs rather than follow a fixed scheme of things set out in any textbook. The Roper model has little sense of priority and the examples in the literature seem to assess the patient always in the same arbitrary order and set out care accordingly. Nurses who intend using Roper should therefore avoid using the standard sequence of headings set out in the model as their order is arbitrary and fails to bring a sense of priority to both assessment and care planning.

The FANCAP scheme is the only assessment to highlight pain as a heading in its own right, although Roy's notion of assessing regulation brings the nurse to an assessment of pain via the nervous system. The other two models require the nurse to assess pain under a specific physiological system; thus, John Harper's pain (Orem) is assessed under aeration and pain for Jenny Haynes (Roper) is mentioned under mobilizing. The two-level assessment of Roy requires the nurse to probe for various reasons other than the obvious that may lie behind the pain. This led to the discovery that Mrs Hill was suffering pain post-operatively not only because of surgery but also because she was very anxious and because she was reluctant to ask for analgesia as she felt this to be a sign of weakness; she was also worried about becoming addicted.

Roper's assessment focuses the nurse's attention on what the patient could do before coming into hospital. However, in acute settings the nurse needs to assess the situation here and now. Home activity and pre-hospital problems are important, but in caring for an acutely ill patient the nurse needs to know the current problems. Time spent on investigating pre-hospital activity needs to be carefully allocated to make sure only relevant information is gathered. Roper's emphasis on 'normal routines' to use her own words may sidetrack the nurse away from important information. There are other issues here, what does normal mean? Normal for whom? What is a routine? How often does something have to be done to be routine? How important is routine? What of the danger of stereotyping the individual and losing their individuality in a grey cloak of conformist, normal routines?

The emphasis of the other models on the here and now is a strength, although the nurse must not lose track of what goes on at home as it may be equally important. However, we should avoid the trap of trying to reduce patients to collections of routines: patients are people not automatons.

There are some areas that do not fit easily into the various assessment schemes of these models. Consider the wound of a patient who has had surgery: it is an obvious feature and a key aspect of post-op care, yet where do these models ask the nurse to assess the wound? The most likely candidate in Orem is the heading 'health deviancy' for that is what a wound is, while the FANCAP heading 'communication' can be interpreted in that way for a wound provides communication between the inside and outside of the body in the same way that the M4 provides communication between London and Bristol. In the Roy and Roper schemes the best that can be suggested is to consider the physiological system relevant to the wound. Thus, a patient who has had gastric surgery might have the wound assessed under nutrition or under eating and drinking, while the bowel surgery undergone by Margaret Hill leads to an assessment under elimination. Roy, though, does have the great advantage of ensuring that the nurse assesses how the patient feels about a wound under the notion of self-concept.

In designing a standard care plan with Roy's model, the nurse does not know which system or area of the body has been affected by the surgery, so an alternative approach is to consider wounds under the oxygenation and circulation part of the assessment on the assumption that, wherever a wound is, it is of significance for the circulation.

A similar problem is encountered with the notion of cleanliness and the condition of a patient's skin. Roper does require an assessment of personal cleansing and dressing — but note the limitations imposed by such terminology as 'normal routines'. This explicit statement about personal hygiene is, however, welcome. The most reasonable approach with another model might be to consider rest and activity (Roy, Orem) or just activity (FANCAP) and assess the patient's activity with regard to personal hygiene. Some nurses, though, might advocate assessing hygiene under elimination. As in the case of wounds, this flexibility is perhaps not a bad thing, but staff should reach a consensus on how they use a model's assessment scheme to ensure there is a degree of consistency in the way it is applied in order to avoid confusion, particularly among students and staff new to the model.

The use of Roy's model would require an assessment of the person's ability to adapt to their condition in pursuit of personal hygiene, while Orem directs the nurse to look at self-care ability. These seem slightly safer concepts than normal routines. Pressure-area risks can be calculated using a standard scale such as Norton or Waterlow and seem relevant when investigating the patient's ability to move about (rest and activity, mobilizing, etc.).

In writing care plans, nurses sometimes have difficulty dealing with the effects of medical interventions such as wound drains and IVIs. Such equipment presents real problems to the patient which must figure in the nursing care, but the question arises of how to incorporate essentially medical interventions into a nursing care plan. The solution requires the nurse to look beyond the IVI or wound drain and ask why it is there? The answer to that question is the real patient problem, i.e. the patient is unable to maintain hydration via the oral route (IVI) or an accumulation of serosanguinous fluid may delay wound healing and become infected (wound drain). The patient's problem is then an inability to maintain hydration or the risk of delayed wound healing with typical goals being a fluid intake of 3L/day or that the wound will heal without any complications within 14 days. The care of the IVI or wound drain then logically becomes a nursing intervention.

Invasive medical interventions such as these can be seen within the Roy model as maladaptive in so far as they breach our normal defences against infection (the integrity of the skin), while from Orem's point of view they represent self-care deficits in that the patient cannot prevent the possibility of infection occurring at the site of insertion. The risk of infection then becomes a potential patient problem.

Human physiology is a very closely integrated collection of systems which has to achieve balance or homeostasis for healthy functioning. For this reason it seems better to bring together notions of input and output and assess them together as they affect a bodily system, since one very much depends on the other. For this reason the four Orem headings of intake of air, water and food plus elimination have been reduced to three — aeration, fluid balance and nutrition, each of which is assessed from the point of view of intake and output (p. 44). This reflects the FANCAP approach and avoids the duplication shown in the Roper assessment of Jenny Haynes. Perhaps the Roper model would benefit from separating the eating and drinking heading into two separate parts, and considering elimination under eating and then again separately under drinking, removing the separate elimination heading from the model.

The notion of assessing pulse separately from blood pressure and respiratory rate in Roper's model seems strange given the above observation. The cardiovascular and respiratory systems are inextricably entwined, survival would not be possible otherwise. Thus, whether it is a heading such as aeration (Orem, FANCAP) or oxygenation and circulation (Roy), both systems must be assessed together and care must be planned in an integrated way. In this way John Harper receives care that ensures there is enough oxygen getting into his arterial blood and that blood plus oxygen is being efficiently pumped around his body. Such an integrated approach is lacking in the arbitrary and disjointed headings used by Roper.

The probems discussed above indicate the need for a flexible and pragmatic approach to the use of nursing models if they are to be translated into the real world of clinical nursing and be recognized as valid tools to enable and facilitate nursing care.

The health deviancy aspect of Orem's model is an interesting concept in that it requires the nurse to look at how the patient is being affected by specific pathology and how well he or she is coping not only with that pathology but also with the effects of the medical treatment that is being given, e.g. knowledge of drugs being taken as in the case of John Harper. Whilst the emphasis on health promotion and independent nursing care are welcome developments, nursing cannot ignore medical practice and illness as they affect the patient, and consequently this aspect of Orem's model is very helpful.

In using Roy the nurse must be prepared to apply the concept of pathology and treatment to the specific systems of the body in turn, as there is no specific 'health deviancy' heading. If John Harper's care were planned using the Roy model, then his lack of knowledge about drug therapy would have to be assessed under the heading oxygenation and circulation. In using the Roper model the nurse might choose to make such assessments under the heading of maintaining a safe environment, a heading which, however, overlaps considerably with 'mobility'.

The important psychosocial aspects of care figure prominently in the Roy model with the notions of self-concept, role function and interdependence. Consideration of the two care plans, however, reveals that role function and interdependence are very closely related. Margaret Hill's role as a mother is bound up with her feelings about the independence of her children. At present she has no sexual partner, being recently widowed; however, if she did, consider how personal and physical self-concept after colostomy might interact with her role as a sexual partner, lover and wife, which in turn would affect her interdependence with her partner. It seems as though these three psychosocial areas of behaviour and adaptation are different but overlapping ways of looking at the same field. By analogy, to appreciate what any object looks like, a person must look at it from different points of view to see it in three dimensions. Inevitably view A will partly look the same as view B, but view B will contain new information not seen in view A and so on for view C. In the same way, self-concept, role function and interdependence describe a whole range of aspects of a person's psychosocial functioning, inevitably with some degree of overlap because of the complexity of the ways humans think and behave.

Orem's model places emphasis on how the patient relates to others in assessing 'solitude-socialization' and the admittedly vague concept of 'normalcy' can be interpreted in terms of how anxious is the patient feeling about the situation he is in or likely to be in. It is important that such a vague term has an agreed common meaning for all the staff using the model if consistency of assessment and hence care is to be achieved.

The developmental component of Orem's model is a strong tool for assessing how patients are managing to cope with their stage in the life cycle. Roy's interdependence, role function and personal self-concept modes can be used to arrive at similar information, providing the nurse is sensitive to the notion of the patient moving along a life continuum of constant change associated with ageing. The views expressed by Mabel Bush in the Orem developmental assessment could be interpreted as an elderly lady with no relatives (interdependence) who feels she has outlived her usefulness and has no purpose left in life (role function), having such a low self-esteem that she just wants to die (personal self-concept). Her isolation is confirmed from the 'socialization' heading, while we note from 'normalcy' that she misses her husband badly.

The Orem model can therefore be used to assess and plan for similar dimensions of psychosocial care as Roy, although there is a different emphasis, self-care as opposed to adaptation. The question remains whether it is better to talk of self-care or adaptation in, for example, coming to terms with widowhood. Perhaps such ideas are so closely linked that they cannot be separated in practice, for to adapt the woman has to be self-reliant (self-caring), yet to be self caring she needs to have reconciled herself to her bereavement and carried out the necessary grief work — that is, to be self-caring she has to adapt.

The FANCAP scheme is more concerned with urgent physiological problems, although a heading such as communication does open up a wide field of investigation, as through communication the nurse can learn a great deal about the patient's fears and anxieties. The assessments of Darren Mardon and Patrick Dunne both contain reference under fluids to family and friends. This may seem a little puzzling, however it is suggested that as fluids possess a property called fluidity, this property might legitimately be included in the assessment. Fluidity corresponds to an absence of friction and may therefore be interpreted as how well does the patient get along with people, what are his social networks? If the nurse wishes to extend the FANCAP scheme in this way, the notion of activity might be taken to include work and recreational activity, allowing for the inclusion of further important social information about the patient and directing the care planner to think in terms of how for example, Darren, will manage in his job after this accident and whether he will be able to continue playing competitive football.

The Roper model fails to get to grips with the richness and complexity of the way humans think and behave; the intricately woven tapestry of psychological and social activity is reduced to a polaroid snapshot in this model. The model lacks any serious attempt to understand how the patient is feeling, what their background is, why they do the things they do. Instead there is an arbitrary and disjointed checklist of physical aspects of behaviour. How does Mrs Haynes feel about being elderly, possibly having to be cared for by her younger sister who she cannot get on with and has never liked? Her loss of independence has been greatly worrying her, and now comes this stroke on top of everything else. She hates herself for not being able to get to the toilet in time; it is so childish to be incontinent so she will not drink much, leading to dehydration. She used to be a very active women, but now age has made her feel sad and useless, forced to live with a younger sister she has never liked. None of this information is likely to come out of a Roper-style assessment consisting of noting how well she could walk or cook at home before her illness.

Consider Bill Slater, an ex-publican who has a significant alcohol problem. So much might be suspected from the Roper assessment, but that is all. A different approach might have revealed that he hates being at home, has major problems in getting on with his wife, and spends most of his time in the pub. He continues to smoke despite his COAD because he believes that having a good cough helps clear his chest and smoking also calms his nerves; he is unaware just how smoky an environment a pub is because he has worked in one for so long. Information such as that might have been derived from the Roy two-level assessment approach, which is lacking in Roper. Bill spends a lot of time in the pub because that is where his friends are, the old regulars; they give him a social life he does not have elsewhere. He also has a degree of prestige as the ex-landlord that is good for his self-esteem. He cannot adjust to being retired as he feels useless, and this makes him unhappy. He gets under his wife's feet at home so they have rows and he goes to the pub to get out of the way, while their sex life fizzled out many years ago.

Bill Slater, therefore has, a fundamentally unhealthy lifestyle related to social and psychological problems. As long as he is drinking and smoking heavily, eating a poor diet and spending a lot of time in the pub, he will be prone to increasingly worse attacks of COAD, becoming severely restricted in his mobility, and at increasing risk of alcohol-related accidents and pathology, not to mention heart disease. The Orem/Roy approach is more likely to get to the root of these problems than the Roper checklist, which might only ensure that the basics of physical care are attempted by nursing staff while he is in hospital. The word 'attempted' has been chosen deliberately as Bill may well respond with hostility to having his life organized by nurses, leading to non-compliance and the 'difficult patient' label. Bill's problems are of the chronic type, which were discussed on p. 37 where it was shown that self-care and self-concept were crucial in successful management and reducing the problem of non-compliance. An interactionist perspective may show his apparent non-compliance in a new light when he is considered as a man who has been independent all his life and who is now losing that independence owing to retirement. However, it needs an approach to nursing that will explore these psychosocial areas in a way that Roper does not, to shed that light upon the patient.

In order to have effective care, the patient must be working with the nurse. An approach to nursing that explores the psychosocial aspects of a patient is more likely to succeed in this goal as it allows the nurse to begin to see the reasons why the patient is behaving the way he or she is. Roper's physical task checklist does not provide a framework for that degree of understanding.

If we consider again the four basic components of any model — the person, environment, health and nursing — Roper's model fragments the person into arbitrary physiological systems, ignores the social, psychological and environmental components of life, and presents health in a negative way that leads to a focus on ill-health and patient labelling. In the light of such an unhappy performance on the first three components, it is not surprising to find the model leading to a simplistic approach to nursing that fails to recognize the patient as an integrated person.

In conclusion, the above discussion suggests that the Roper model of nursing has major weaknesses as a model upon which to base general hospital care when compared to other alternatives. Reference to the criteria on p. 53 for the ideal hospital model show that it also fails to pass most of these tests, succeeding only in being simple and in recognizing the need for the patient to function at home. Roy is perhaps stronger than Orem in showing the patient to be an integrated human being, but Orem has the advantage of stressing developmental effects and also health education. The FANCAP scheme meets some of these criteria, particularly in very acute, high-dependency situations. All models need using with the patient's point of view in mind.

There is sufficient merit in the work of Orem, Roy and also the FANCAP assessment scheme to suggest that they should be developed further in hospital care, being either refined, adapted or even partly merged. The Roper model, however, has such serious flaws that, while the underlying concept of independence is of value, the current approach should be radically reworked or abandoned in favour of more patient-sensitive models of care.

References

Black D *et al.* (1981) *Inequalities in Health*. London: Penguin.

Whithead M (1987) *The Health Divide*. London: Penguin.

5 MODELS IN COMMUNITY CARE

Introduction

The whole area of community care and its method of delivery is going through a period of uncertainty and change as a result of the legislative changes brought about by government. What is not changing, however, is the need for community care by many patients, an increasing number of whom are elderly and frail. The community nursing services are fundamental to caring for patients outside hospital and therefore the notion of nursing models is just as important and relevant to community nursing as to hospital based nursing. However, it is important that models are not seen as panaceas that will resolve all community nursing's problems, for they will not. If treated in that superficial and unrealistic way they are only likely to add to the lengthening list of problems that community care faces today.

In this chapter the differing nature of the care environment will be explored to consider what implications this has for nursing models, and then we will consider the care of several of the patients encountered in the previous chapter after discharge.

Characteristics needed for models in community care

Community nurses are very busy people and could be forgiven for thinking that models are all about theorizing, which is all very well for those who have the time, but the average community nurse has to get on with caring for patients. Consequently, models may seem of little value to community nurses. As nurses build up their experience in caring for patients at home, they might also feel that they develop an intuitive feeling for the care that is required. Nursing models may therefore be seen as a rigid bureaucratic approach to care that interferes with the nurse's own experience-based view of how an individual should be nursed. If a model is to avoid rejection on these grounds it needs flexibility and it has to be seen as something that helps rather than hinders.

This view corresponds with the description of the 'expert nurse' given by Benner (1984), who suggests that this is the final stage of development reached by nurses as they evolve from being novices to advanced beginners, competent and then proficient practitioners. Benner discusses the need for frameworks and guidance to help the nurse reach the expert stage and it could therefore be argued that the use of nursing models at least in the early stages of a community nurse's career, helps to achieve the later stages of proficiency and expertise. The hospital nurse works in an environment where there are usually other nurses to turn to for help and advice; the community nurse, although part of a team, spends much of his or her time with patients alone. Hence the need for a framework to assist the nurse along Benner's road to expertise. That framework is a nursing model.

In discussing nurses' own informal models of care, Luker (1988) commented on how important they are in pointing the direction that individual nurses are likely to follow in carrying out care but also noted that they tend to lead to an informal and unsystematic way of working which she considered characteristic of many community nurses. Luker went on to point out that it is very difficult to share such informal models of care with others.

When this is considered in conjunction with the often single-handed nature of the community nurse's work, and Benner's analysis of how nursing expertise develops, an argument in favour of nursing models starts to emerge. It is essential, given the different members of the community team who may visit the patient at home, that everybody is using the same approach to care. Care must be consistent and not contradictory as different members of the nursing team visit the patient. This emphasizes the need for a harmonized approach to care, with all members of the community nursing team using an agreed common model of nursing.

Such a model for the community needs to reflect the experiences of many different practitioners and their patients, allowing nurses to structure care in a logical way that is easily shared with others. The model therefore needs to be based in reality and be derived from that reality. It needs to be as unambiguous as possible — jargon is positively harmful in this respect.

Community care involves the patient (and family) dealing with his or her own health care needs. This leads towards a philosophy of self-care or independence. It is essential for continuity of care that the approach of the family and patient should reflect the philosophy of the nurse. In order to achieve such harmonization, a simple model that is readily grasped by lay carers is essential. Simplicity and a focus on independence therefore emerge as key ingredients of any community model.

A nursing approach that is aiming at self-care or independence can, however, be misinterpreted by the patient or family as neglect or a lack of care. There is a thin dividing line between the nurse saying 'You must learn to do this for yourself Mrs Smith' and the perception that this is because the nurse cannot be bothered to do whatever it is for Mrs Smith herself. This points to the need for an open discussion about the main aims of care with the patient and family so that the model or philosophy of care is fully understood.

The model may, however, be rejected by the patient, which leaves the nurse in a difficult position, being very much a guest in the patient's home, seeing the patient perhaps for half an hour every other day. Tactful negotiation and compromise, coupled with recognition of the patient's own rights of self determination are essential in this situation.

The involvement of the family in care, and the recognition that such care is carried out in the home requires that any model should address the importance of family relationships and other social factors relevant to the patient's domestic situation. Unless the model directs the nurse to assess such areas and formulate goals that are appropriate, it is of little value in community nursing.

The patient discharged from hospital may have received very variable amounts of discharge information and health education. Ever-earlier discharges reduce the amount of time available for ward-based patient teaching. The community nurse, therefore, can usually expect that patients will need a substantial amount of teaching and education in the immediate short term after discharge, followed by encouragement and reinforcement to sustain health-oriented interventions such as dieting, giving up smoking or reducing alcohol intake over a prolonged period of time. A strong health education component is therefore seen as an essential ingredient of a successful community model of nursing care.

Continuity of care requires that just as the family and community nurse should try to harmonize their care philosophy, so too should the hospital and community team. A nursing model that is to be applied in the community should ideally be the same as that used in hospital in order to avoid the confusion that may follow in the patient's own mind on seeing the nursing care given after discharge contradicting the care given in hospital. It may be argued that the environment and health status of the patient after discharge are very different from in hospital and that, therefore, it is inappropriate to try to use the same model of care. In many cases, however, a change in emphasis or in the way the model is interpreted can accommodate this change. Orem's model is particularly striking in this respect as the model has the built-in notion of different systems of nursing care which reflect the whole continuum of dependency.

This requires of models that they be flexible enough to apply equally well in hospital and community settings, but it also requires nurses to be flexible and creative in the way that they use models if this goal is to be achieved. A piece of rubber is very flexible, but only if a person bothers to try to bend it; so too with a nursing model, even if it is flexible, it will only meet the patient's needs if the nurse has the wit to utilize it individually and creatively.

However, if the nurse feels that a change of model is justified upon discharge, it is important to discuss this change in philosophy with the patient in order that the patient fully understands the changes which may occur in care and the reasons behind such changes.

Community nurses therefore need a common repertoire of nursing models shared with their hospital colleagues in order that the care required for differing patients after discharge may be continued without any major hiatus or contradiction. Hospital and community nurses need to discuss models and arrive at an agreed range of models that will commonly be used in both care environments.

The basic requirements of nursing models that are applicable to community care can therefore be summarized as follows.

(1) They must be simple, flexible and jargon free if implementation is to be realistically expected in the busy community environment.
(2) Any model must be rooted in the shared experience of other community nurses if it is to help beginners achieve expertise.
(3) The importance of family and social networks must be emphasized.
(4) The philosophy of the model should reflect the real world of the patient having to care for him/herself therefore notions of independence and self-care should figure prominently.
(5) Continuity of care is best achieved if the model is the same as that which was used in hospital care. The emphasis and interpretation may differ, however, in the differing circumstances and on occasion a complete change in approach may be felt valid.
(6) Health education and long-term support must figure prominently.

In the following care plans, some of the patients encountered in the previous chapter will be studied in their home environments to see how the models used to plan care in hospital may be extended into the community setting. How well they measure up against the above criteria will be considered at the end of the chapter.

Jenny Haynes and the Roper Model

In the previous chapter we saw how the Roper model could be used to construct a plan of care for this 78-year-old lady who had been admitted to hospital after suffering a CVA. The next step will be to look at how a community nurse might use Roper to plan care for this lady after discharge.

Continuity of care was discussed in the preceding section and in the interests of achieving this goal we will hypothesize that a copy of the patient's hospital nursing care plan (p. 79) has accompanied her home. This would allow the community nurse to immediately note the patient's level of independence in the various ADLs prior to her CVA without lengthy questioning. The hospital admission assessment also gives the community nurse a baseline to work from, as it should show how much progress has been made by the patient in recovering independence.

The following care plan has been derived therefore from comparing the level of independence demonstrated by the patient upon returning home with the usual independent routines outlined in the hospital assessment in order to discover problems. The plan is by no means exhaustive, rather it is a sample of the sort of problems that may be taken as representative of such a patient when the Roper model is applied in this context. Clearly this plan will change with time as frequent reassessment of the progress being made by the patient occurs.

Care plan: Jenny Haynes

Problem	Goal	Intervention
(1) Access to bath/bedroom limited by risk of falling on stairs due to L-sided weakness (A).	Pt will toilet and sleep downstairs.	1. Rearrange furniture downstairs. 2. Order commode.
	Pt will return to use of bed/bathroom (L).	1. OT Assessment for stair handrail. 2. Encourage physio at day hospital.
(2) Anxious about stairs due to L-side weakness (A).	Pt will state less anxious about falling.	1. Let Pt talk about fears. 2. See above.
(3) Slurring of speech persists (A).	Pt will improve verbal communication.	1. Listen carefully. 2. Encourage speech. 3. Discuss with Pt's sister. 4. Arrange Speech Therapist appt.
(4) Discharge Wt 73 kg Ht 5ft 0in. Obesity therefore restricting movement (A).	Pt to lose 8 kg in 3 months.	1. Discuss diet with Pt and sister. 2. Give reducing diet sheets.
(5) Reluctance to drink due to fear of incontinence may lead to dehydration.	Fluid intake of at least 2L/day.	1. Explain importance of drinking; see (7). 2. Maintain fluid chart as reminder.
(6) Constipation (A).	Pt will have bowels open every 2 days.	1. (4) 1, (4) 2 above to include fibre. 2. See (5) above. 3. Mild aperient prn.
(7) Incontinence of urine (A).	Pt will not be incontinent.	1. Order commode for downstairs. 2. Pelvic floor exercises. 3. Reduce fluid intake in evening; see (5).
(8) Unable to maintain personal hygiene (A).	Pt will state she is happy with personal hygiene.	1. Arrange 3 baths/wk with DN. 2. Strip wash with help of sister ×4/wk.

Problem	Goal	Intervention
		3. Deliver bath board and seat.
		4. Encourage maximum Pt participation.
(9) Unable to dress self (A).	Pt will be able to dress unaided in 1 month.	1. Reinforce and encourage skills learnt in hospital.
		2. Discuss clothing adaptation, e.g. Velcro.
(10) Hypothermia (P).	Pt will not develop hypothermia.	1. Teach Pt & sister.
		2. Give leaflets, etc.
		3. Wall thermometer.
		4. Refer Social Worker re benefits.
(11) Restricted mobility. Cannot walk without another person to help (A).	Will be able to walk 20 m with walking aid only.	1. Day hosp. physio.
		2. Teach passive exercises to Pt & sister.
		3. Encouragement and practice each visit.
(12) Pressure sores (P).	Pt will not develop any pressure sores.	1. Teach Pt & sister about pressure care; devise care plan.
(13) Restricted activity may lead to boredom and frustration (P).	Pt will develop new interests.	1. Provide wheelchair.
		2. Son-in-law to build ramp to front door.
		3. Refer to voluntary community visitors.
		4. Contact local day centre, arrange transport.
		5. Explore potential skills with OT.
(14) Difficulty in sleeping downstairs (A).	Pt will have min. of 7 hours sleep/night.	1. Hospital medication to continue in reduced dose.
		2. Review in 1 week.
(15) Pt stated 'I would have been better off dead'. Depressed (A).	Pt will talk positively about the present and tomorrow.	1. Allow PT chance to verbalize fears and anxieties.

The Roy model and Margaret Hill

In the preceding chapter the Roy model was used to plan care for Mrs Hill after she had undergone bowel resection due to cancer and the formation of a colostomy. If a copy of her hospital care plan was sent to the community nurse this would facilitate care by allowing the community nurse to see how Mrs Hill felt about her surgery and how well she adapted in hospital. The assessment follows the convention of identifying what Roy calls 'maladaptive behaviour' by underlining it, in order that problem statements may be formulated reflecting these areas.

First-level assessment	Second-level assessment		
	Focal	Contextual	Residual

PHYSIOLOGICAL MODE

Oxygenation: RR 16, P 74. Non-smoker, no cough.

Fluid balance: Drinking freely, looks well hydrated.

Nutrition: Ht 5ft 5in Wt 45 kg.

	Focal	Contextual	Residual
Lost 5 kg since surgery.	Surgery		
Anxious and uncertain about diet, eating little.	Lacks knowledge of what to eat.	Dislikes stoma func-tioning.	Worried bag will leak.

Elimination: Stoma is pink, looks healthy, functioning 2–3 times/day. Pt unhappy about changing bag.

	Focal	Contextual	Residual
	Disgust at contents.	Dislikes smell in house.	Afraid 'may catch something'.
Abdominal wound healed but has discharging sinus.	Wound infection.		
Frequency and pain on PU.	UTI.		
Rest/exercise: Sleeping very poorly.	Anxiety.	Afraid bag will leak in her bed.	
Feels fatigued.	Major surgery.	Anaemic.	
Regulation: Still has some pain and discomfort.	Surgery.		

SELF-CONCEPT MODE

	Focal	Contextual	Residual
Physical: Disgusted at the stoma. 'Thought I could cope as it was only temporary, but it's so horrible'.	Appearance of stoma.		Beliefs about normal bowel function.
Worried about weight loss.	Loss of 10 kg in 4 months.	Clothes lost fit and shape.	Belief it's a bad sign.
Personal: Feels worthless and power-less.	Stoma.	Loss of control over body function.	Afraid to meet people ashamed of stoma.
Fears the cancer may return.	Knows surgery was for cancer.		'You can't cure cancer, it kills you in the end'.

ROLE FUNCTION MODE

	Focal	Contextual	Residual
Anxious about returning to work, loss of income.	Surgery will mean off work for 4–6 weeks.	How will others at work accept her stoma?	
Worried stoma will stop her enjoying grandchildren. Isolation from family.	Fears she cannot play with them.		Fears family may reject her now.

INTERDEPENDENCY MODE

	Focal	Contextual	Residual
Depressed about future relationships.	Fears nobody will want to know her with stoma.		
Fears will lose independence if cancer returns.	Knows diagnosis.		Belief cancer will return.

Mabel Bush and the Orem self-care model

Mabel was discharged home two weeks after surgery, still in need of a significant amount of nursing care. Her self-care ability needs to be examined in the light of her pre-hospital, as well as her present, abilities. Discharge home with a copy of her hospital care plan for the community nurse will greatly facilitate this process and in constructing this assessment and care plan it will be assumed that this was the case. The community nurse therefore already has a baseline of her pre-illness self-care ability to work from (p. 60).

Post-discharge self-care ability

AERATION	Very SOB on exertion, cannot manage steps. P 88 irreg., RR 22.
FLUID BALANCE	Remains anxious about incontinence and is reluctant to drink. Admits she had several 'accidents' in hospital.
NUTRITION	Cannot now get to the shops and admits to still being worried about her constipation. Can cook for herself although preparing some food will be difficult (e.g. vegetables).
ACTIVITY AND REST	Lacks confidence in walking, can only manage a few yards with the aid of a stick. Admits she is frightened of what will happen to her if she falls over again. Cannot manage steps (see aeration). Sleeping is only possible if she is sat upright as she gets breathless; tends to prefer dozing in a chair. Hopes she can resume her embroidery. Is aware that she cannot now manage to bath herself or use the bathroom. There is a pressure sore on the back of her R. heel, dressed with Opsite.
SOCIALIZATION/SOLITUDE	Is very concerned about being a burden on her neighbour. Does not think family will be bothered with her; fearful of living alone and how she will manage the house.
HAZARDS	Feels she may fall again; worried about security of house with her on her own inside.
NORMALCY	Relieved to be out of hospital, acknowledges everybody was very kind and helpful, but did not like it there. Glad to be home, but unsure of the future now, feeling sad and wondering what will happen to her. Is thinking about selling up and moving to a nursing home, but she and her husband had lived in this house for nearly 50 years so she is very reluctant to do so.
DEVELOPMENTAL	'My body is letting me down, you get so useless when you are old'. Mabel seems depressed and unable to carry on with life alone, feels this is the beginning of the end. (See admission assessment).
HEALTH DEVIANCY	Remains uncertain about her medication. Her hip is still painful and there is some ankle oedema, she is sitting with her feet on a foot stool with the pressure over the back of her heels, including the area that has a pressure sore dressing. Is unaware of the cause of her pressure sore. Does not know how she will adapt to her reduced mobility as she does not think she will be able to ever get out of the house again or walk more than a few yards.

By putting together information contained in the hospital care plan and knowledge gained from the above assessment, the community nurse may devise a plan of care similar to that given below. The whole strategy is centred around improving Mabel's self-care abilities and developing the nursing role away from a largely partially compensatory mode towards a more educative consultative mode.

Self-care deficit (Problem)	*Goal*	*Intervention*
(1) Unable to prevent pressure sore formation (P).	Pt will avoid pressure sore formation.	1. Teach about P.sores. 2. Encourage mobility. 3. Spenco cushion L. heel. 4. Sit on settee, or teach correct use of foot stool.
(2) Uninfected pressure sore R. heel 3 cm diameter.	Sore will heal within 3/12.	1. Granuflex dressing. 2. See (1).

Self-care deficit (Problem)	Goal	Intervention
(3) Unable to maintain own hygiene.	Will be able to carry out own hygiene to a standard acceptable to Pt.	1. Order commode, discuss emptying with neighbour. 2. Work out strip-wash routine with Pt. 3. Daily visits to help with (3)2 but encouraging more self-care per visit.
(4) Occasionally unable to maintain continence of urine.	Pt will be continent at all times.	1. Teach pelvic floor exercises. 2. Review diuretic regime teach Pt re diuretics. 3. Pt to keep own fluid chart. See (3) & (9).
(5) Inadequate diet due to lack of knowledge and Pt's inability to shop for self.	Pt to eat healthy well-balanced diet.	1. Discuss difficulties in food preparation. 2. Teach about healthy diet and food prep. 3. Give leaflets on diet. 4. Refer for meals on wheels assessment. 5. Discuss shopping with neighbour.
(6) Pt unable to have normal bowel motions due to constipation (P).	Pt will have bowels open every 2 days.	1. See (5). 2. Fluid intake 2.5L/day; see (4)3. 3. Mild aperients prn.
(7) Pt is unable to maintain social contact (A) which may lead to loneliness and possible disorientation (P).	Pt will engage in social contact and comment favourably on this.	1. Suggest friends visit. 2. Discuss referral to Help the Aged voluntary visitors and luncheon club. 3. Discuss news/current affairs on visits. 4. See (11)3.
(8) Pt does not understand her medication.	Pt will achieve self-medication and show safe level of knowledge of her drugs.	1. Discuss and teach. 2. Measure out daily needs in labelled egg cups. 3. Reinforce importance of medication at each visit. 4. Suggest purchase of tablet dispensing aid.
(9) Pt unable to walk > 7 yds due to fear of falling, pain and SOB (A).	Pt will be able to walk 20 yds, with stick, in 4/52. Short term: 10 yds 1/52, 15 yds 2/52, 15 yds outdoors at 3/52.	1. Discuss how Pt feels about her walking. 2. Encourage walking at each visit, give +ve reinforcement. 3. Check correct use of walking stick. 4. Check safety of floor coverings, furniture, etc. 5. Refer domestic physio? 6. See probs. (7) & (10).
(10) Pt has pain in hips which she cannot relieve (A).	Pt will be able to relieve any pain herself. Pain free in 5/7.	1. Review analgesia with GP. 2. Teach about analgesia. 3. See (8)2. 4. Check positioning for comfort. 5. See (11).

Self-care deficit (Problem)	Goal	Intervention
(11) Pt very anxious about how she will cope on her own (A).	Pt will talk of future plans in a positive way, state less anxious in 2/52.	1. Encourage Pt to talk of worries and how she sees the future. 2. Help Pt explore possible strategies for future. 3. Encourage contact with son living in UK. 4. Check security of house, arrange visit from crime prevention officer. 5. Refer Social Worker. 6. See (7).
(12) Pt may become demoralized and neglect herself (P).	Pt will achieve maximum self-care and express a +ve view of the future.	1. See (7) & (11). 2. Give +ve reinforcement and encouragement for all self-care. 3. Monitor appearance of Pt and house.

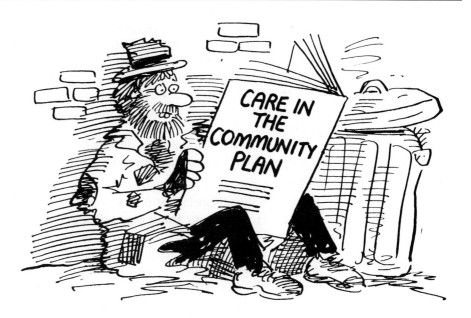

Discussion The experienced community nurse will be aware that there are many social networks supporting the patient at home, some obvious and some not so obvious. These range from immediate family through to neighbours and on to people such as sympathetic local traders, e.g. the milkman or owner of the corner shop. The patient's survival and level of functioning may depend heavily on such networks; it is therefore appropriate to consider how the three models reviewed here treated such networks.

The Roper model, focusing as it does on physiological aspects of independence, clearly failed to point the nurse in the direction of the patient's social networks, which remained largely unexplored in the case of Jenny Haynes. On the other hand, Roy's assessment looked into interdependence and role function and in the case of Margaret Hill allowed the nurse to explore these areas, outlining a variety of problems and possible interventions. By the same token, Orem required the nurse to assess solitude/socialization, which brought out Mabel Bush's fears of becoming a burden and her concern that her family would no longer be bothered with her.

The experienced community nurse using Roper's model may well enquire into such areas automatically, but this should not be taken for granted. Roper's failure to explore social networks compared to the explicit way these areas are to be assessed when using Roy or Orem is unsatisfactory if this model is to be used in the community.

Closely allied with social aspects of care is the question of how patients feel about their problems, what are their fears and anxieties? The psychological dimension of the patient must be considered, and here again we find Roper deficient as there is a lack of room in the assessment to explore feelings. Jenny Haynes stated that she felt she would be better off dead, a chance remark that arose because Roper requires the nurse to explore the patient's views about dying. Setting aside the difficulty of broaching such a subject to a patient, we have only the tip of the iceberg in this despairing comment. Does Roper's model offer the nurse any help in dealing with a patient expressing such views? Could another approach to Jenny Haynes have led the nurse in through easier ground to explore her psychological problems?

Consider the following differing avenues offered by Orem that might permit a gradual opening up of the patient's problems.

(1) 'How easy is it going to be to meet people from now on?' (Solitude/socialization)
(2) 'How do you think you will be able to manage on your own?' (Hazards)
(3) 'What are your feelings about going to a day centre once a week to meet others?' (Normalization)
(4) 'How do you feel your life is changing now?' (Developmental)

Somehow this seems a less direct and confrontational way in to the patient's problems and the philosophy of a continuum of self-care/dependent care gives the nurse some clear ideas to use in trying to develop interventions to meet the patient's needs as they unfurl within this assessment framework. Roy's model might also offer a more perceptive and gradual approach to Jennie's psychological problems, as the nurse can explore how she feels about herself and her relationships with others via the psychosocial modes of the assessment. The care plans for both Margaret Hill and Mabel Bush show a more sensitive and perceptive approach to the patient's psychological problems because the relevant models open the subject area up gradually in the assessment stage and give the nurse a clear and relevant philosophy to work with in planning care.

This difference of approach poses questions such as how well-qualified the nurse is to use the model and whether the nurse has the time and skills to utilize the assessment tool fully. Taking the second question first, it is apparent that Orem and Roy's assessments require the nurse to have considerable skills in questioning in order that various sensitive areas may be explored. Time is also at a premium. Margaret Hill's ability to cope with her stoma is going to depend upon a lot more than mastering the simple mechanical skills of changing a bag, and to help her nursing as a profession must recognize this crucial fact and begin to tackle these difficult areas with tools that are sensitive enough to do the job. Nursing, therefore, will need to develop considerable sophistication if models such as these are to be used in preference to the rather simplistic and naive approach of Roper.

The issue of how the nurse's view of patient problems differs from the patient's is nicely illustrated by Mabel Bush. The nurse sees occasional incontinence as a problem and hopefully sets a goal of trying to minimize accidents in the short term and aiming for a completely dry patient in the long term. However, Mabel might be unconcerned by the odd bit of dampness 'After all I've been through, it's a minor thing' and not see incontinence as a problem. Alternatively, she might cope with the problem by denial, hence the importance of the community nurse using all her senses in assessing a patient. The unmistakable odour of incontinence might have to be reconciled with a patient steadily denying having any problems. Jenny Haynes may view her house as adequately heated, having become unaware of the real cold, and may consider her weight no problem at all while Margaret Hill may be convinced, despite all assurances to the contrary, that her stoma bag smells offensively.

In each of these three patients, it can be seen that, whichever model is used, the patient's perception of a problem may be very different from the nurse's. Unless the nurse is aware of this and is prepared to try to see things from the patient's point of view, then progress will be very limited. All three models used here lack a patient perspective as they were originally formulated and the nurse must be prepared to graft onto these models a notion of the patient's point of view.

In the introduction to this chapter we emphasized the fact that the community nurse is operating as part of a team of carers, and how important it is for all members of that team to share the same philosophy of care. There is little value in the community nurse aiming to make patients as independent as possible or to maximize their self-care ability if other members of the team such as the Nursing Auxiliary or Health Care Assistant carry out all care for the patient at the expense of self-care or independence.

It is easy to see how, in the case of Jenny Haynes, goals and interventions for problems (8) and (9) in the care plan could easily be undermined by a well-intentioned assistant who washed and dressed the patient totally because it was simply quicker than spending the time involved in letting the patient do as much as possible for herself. Similar observations relate to Mabel Bush (e.g. problems (3) and (9)). Unless all the care team and the informal carers of the patient are speaking the same language and sticking to the same plan of care, then chaos and confusion will result, with the patient picking up mixed messages and the district nurse's plans coming to nought, whatever model they are based upon.

It may be argued that Roy's model is the most complex and that therefore it is here that misunderstandings may occur. It is the author's experience in teaching this model that students often disagree whether a stimulus is focal, contextual or residual. Consideration of the nutrition part of Margaret Hill's assessment is a case in point, as it is a matter of opinion whether the prime cause of her eating little is a lack of knowledge (as stated here and therefore the focal stimulus for the problem) or whether it is a dislike of the stoma functioning (here assumed to be a contextual stimulus). If these two causes or stimuli were reversed and her dislike of the stoma functioning was considered to be focal while the lack of knowledge was considered contextual, would it make any difference to the plan of care?

The answer of course is no. What matters is that we have identified a problem — the patient is eating little and is very anxious and uncertain about what she should be eating — and have discovered that this is due to a combination of a lack of knowledge about diet and a dislike of the stoma functioning (and also a fear of the bag leaking, the residual stimulus). Roy's model urges intervention wherever possible around the causes of the problems and that is what the care plan sets out to do by teaching her about her diet and helping her adapt in a variety of ways to the stoma. The title 'focal' and 'contextual' become academic in this context; what matters is that we have identified a problem, worked out the causes of the problem, and are directing nursing care at those causes.

The community nurse should not, therefore, become too preoccupied with the academic minutiae of models, particularly the more complex ones such as Roy, but should adopt a more pragmatic approach to making the general principles work. Having said that, it is still a fact that Roy's model makes the nurse consistently look into the causes of the patient's problems in a way that none of the other models do. To some extent this might leave the nurse guessing at the causes of some problems; there has always been a place in nursing for intuition and the experienced community nurse probably incorporates a significant amount of intuition in his or her day-to-day work anyway. If Roy requires the nurse to use intuition from time to time, then so be it, and no bad thing either.

This chapter would not be complete without acknowledging that access to hospital-based information and care plans for community nurses is often not all that it should be. It has been assumed that the community nurse had access to hospital care plans for the three patients studied in this chapter, a factor which would save a great deal of time if this were standard practice. How the break-up of the NHS that seems likely under the current legislation will affect hospital–community liaison remains to be seen, but the signs are not encouraging. One thing that is clear is that the government's dehumanization of people into 'packages of care' with the emphasis very much on 'social care' emphasizes the need for community nursing care in the future to be very much geared to the social dimensions of the patient, a fact that requires consideration in choosing models of practice.

This discussion leads us to the conclusions that the Roy and Orem models probably have significant advantages over the more physiologically orientated approach of Roper in planning nursing care in the community. However, such advantages are largely hypothetical because, as has been argued elsewhere, there is a dearth of serious research looking at different nursing models in practice. The ideas of Roy and Orem do, however, have much to commend them to the community nurse.

Community nurses may argue that they would like to introduce the sort of innovative change argued for here, but the Health Authority only has standard paperwork based upon one model, usually Roper. Such a single-model approach to nursing is unimaginative in the extreme and as the stultifying effect of over-centralized bureaucracy has been well demonstrated in the USSR today, perhaps nursing too needs its own 'perestroika'. We suggest that the community nurse can take an immediate step in that direction by combining the Health Authority forms with the most simple form of all, a blank piece of paper, to carry out a patient assessment. Further, how the nurse thinks about care is free from paperwork, the nurse's own philosophy of care is not found in a procedure manual.

Combining these two observations, the community nurse who wishes to use the differing approaches of various theorists should not feel constrained by paperwork. The essential extra information required for model implementation can be recorded on a blank piece of paper and the basic ideas that go with using a model are free and in the nurse's own head. Models of nursing are after all primarily ways of thinking about nursing, and no Health Authority General Manager has yet claimed the Orwellian powers of the 'Thought Police'.

References

Benner P (1984) *From Nurse to Expert*, Addison Wesley, Menlo Park.

Luker K (1988) Do Nursing models work? *Nursing Times* 84:5, 27–29.

6 MENTAL HEALTH NURSING AND MODELS

In researching this book, the author was struck by the relative lack of literature on models of nursing in the field of mental health when compared to general nursing. It therefore seems appropriate to explore what has been written, addressing questions such as how appropriate nursing models are in this field, whether they are workable and what general nurses can learn from looking at nursing models in mental health. It is hoped to stimulate debate in these areas and that the reader will see the arguments in the wider context of the whole book.

It is widely acknowledged that a large proportion of the community will probably have mental health problems at some stage in their lives. It is therefore interesting to note that Wilkinson (1988) has pointed out that 95% of these people will NOT see a psychiatrist, but instead have treatment from their GP and a wide range of other professional groups in which nursing figures very prominently. Wilkinson argues that GPs turn increasingly to nurses, social workers, counsellors (who may be nurses) and clinical psychologists to help patients with mental health problems. Various studies (Mangen *et al.*, 1983; Paykel, 1982) have demonstrated clear benefits to patients who were cared for by community psychiatric nurses rather than psychiatrists on an outpatient basis. More recent work in Manchester confirms the view of Rae (1990) that patients treated in day hospitals will have a lower relapse rate than those admitted to hospital as inpatients for treatment of acute episodes of mental illness, although this latter group may show a more rapid short-term improvement.

The continuing policy of discharging patients from mental hospitals to the community will only serve to further increase the already heavy workload of nurses and other professional groups in providing care for the mentally ill. We may see, therefore, that a major component of care for the mentally ill is carried out by nurses, increasingly in the community. The issue of models of nursing is therefore very relevant to mental health care in the 1990s.

Within the field of psychiatry there are already a range of models of mental illness which Collister (1986) feels most nurses are familiar with, listing the medical-biological, behaviourist, psychoanalytical and socio-interpersonal models as four main models. There are various other ways of looking at or modelling mental illness besides these four approaches, which were described by Siegler and Osmond (1966). Differing views of mental illness will lead to differing approaches to therapy, the nurse–patient relationship and a whole range of other variables.

The literature, and also the reality of practice, however, gives less prominence to nursing models of mental health care as the medical model remains in the ascendancy in many areas. Nursing models should not be thought of as alternative models of mental illness to those cited above, but rather as models of caring for patients with a mental illness, however that illness is conceptualized.

Smith (1986) has commented on the fact that doctors hold views, which are often strongly stated, on approaches to medical care, patients and also nurses, while nurses too hold views on doctors, patients and medical care. However, what is lacking from nurses in Smith's view, is a body of knowledge and opinion about psychiatric nursing care, although she hopes that changes in the education of nurses for the mental health part of the Register will rectify this weakness.

The dominance of the medical model, with its reliance on physical treatment and chemotherapy aiming at a cure, has had profound effects on nursing. It is true, though, that some patients present for treatment in such a disturbed condition that drug therapy is needed to stabilize the situation before any further progress in care or therapy can begin. Nurses have frequently tended to work with specific disease labels in institutional settings, with the emphasis often on custodial care. The dehumanizing effects of the large institutions is well known and, as we have seen in general nursing, focusing on a disease leads to losing sight of the whole person. This is the history that mental health nursing has been trying to grow away from in the 1980s.

There are parallels with general nursing; here nurses are trying to establish nursing as a profession independent of medicine with functions other than following doctors' orders. In fairness to the medical profession, it has to be said that they have their point of view as well as nurses, and this can be very imaginative and creative in many cases. The reader should beware stereotyping and those who would reduce medical–nursing relationships to a state of trench warfare! However, an independent profession of mental health nursing requires the creation of a body of professional knowledge and a view of health care that is unique to nursing, hence the growth of nursing models to try to give a theoretical framework to this effort. Inevitably this might lead to differences with other groups of staff who have different views of mental illness and therapeutic models. But an independent profession should be mature enough to handle such potential conflicts and find negotiated solutions.

Just as general nurses are wrestling with the question 'What is nursing?' so too nurses in the field of mental health must tackle this question. General nursing faces the problem of increasing numbers of paramedical and technical staff taking away bits and pieces of care and treatment, leading to the risk of fragmentation of patient care and the deskilling of nursing. The notion of a nursing body of knowledge and nursing models of practice is an attempt to define the boundaries and profession of nursing. Mental health faces similar problems as various professionals such as clinical psychologists, social workers and occupational therapists increasingly take over aspects of patient care, leading to a loss of continuity and the erosion of the nursing role until little more than a custodial function involving meeting basic physiological and safety needs remains. The development of lay advocacy groups acting to protect the patient's interests is a further challenge to the nursing role.

General nursing has learnt a great deal from mental health nursing in terms of seeing the patient as a whole person rather than a piece of pathology (the medical model). It would be ironic if mental health nursing were now to ignore the lessons that general nursing could teach, i.e. the need to define an integrated profession of mental health nursing with its own body of knowledge and models of practice unique to nursing, rather than borrowed from elsewhere. Fitzpatrick *et al.* (1982) have pointed out that nursing's willingness to embrace non-nursing models in psychiatry has done psychiatric nursing a disservice, while McKenna (1989) in a discussion of this issue urges nurses in mental health to strive to develop nursing models of practice rather than rely exclusively on the views of other, different professions. In making this plea, McKenna cites the work of Reed (1987), who argues that only nursing models can lead to a clear understanding of the theoretical and conceptual basis of psychiatric nursing.

If nurses in the field of mental health wish to move once and for all away from the custodial role, then they have to be prepared to move away from the safe ground of the medical model and following doctors' orders to explore new territory, claiming this as mental health nursing. Failure to do so now will mean that in the future most of that territory will have been partitioned out among a wide range of other groups of staff, particularly in the community, leaving mental health nurses as guardians of the keys and the doers of messy jobs that nobody else wants. Welcome initiatives are to be found at present, but do these pioneers carry the majority of mental nurses with them yet? In thinking this issue through, the great shift of patients to the community cannot be ignored, although the Government was forced to withdraw its Community Care Bill in 1990 as the huge resource and organizational difficulties it entailed were finally realized.

Smith (1986) is only one of many authors who has highlighted the traditionally low prestige of mental health nursing, pointing out that the development of a uniquely nursing knowledge base and the use of nursing models as a conceptual framework would be an essential part of a programme aimed at professionalizing this branch of nursing. She goes on, however, to raise the issues of autonomy and accountability. General nurses are becoming increasingly aware of these issues, which have major implications in the field of mental health. Nurses must be prepared to be responsible and hence accountable for their actions if they are to move out from under the medical wing.

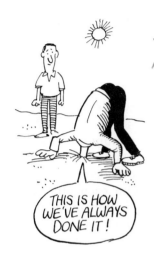

THIS IS HOW WE'VE ALWAYS DONE IT!

It would be unwise in such cases to rely on tradition or an argument such as 'This is the way we have always done it' as the basis for actions for which a nurse is being held accountable. A much stronger rationale is required for safe, expert, professional practice. Walsh and Ford (1989) have written at length about the problems of such unthinking, ritualistic practice in general nursing and it seems that mental health nursing might also have its fair share of rituals and myths. The arguments around autonomy and accountability lead directly to the need for a sound nursing knowledge base.

The discussion so far leads to the conclusion that mental health nursing faces a choice. If it wishes to develop a professional identity of its own, which should benefit both clients and practitioners, then there is a need to develop a unique body of knowledge of which nursing models would form a key part. The phrase mental *health* nursing is chosen quite deliberately, as another prime factor would be an emphasis upon health rather than illness in such a nursing approach. An alternative choice is to continue as before, making the best of other people's views of mental illness, such as the medical models, but aware of the possible retrograde steps towards a deskilled, custodially oriented labour force this may involve.

In the next section of this chapter, models of nursing and some of their basic characteristics will be reviewed to see which most lend themselves towards use in the field of mental health.

Discussion elsewhere has identified that models of nursing contain four basic components: a view of the person, how that person reacts with their environment, an understanding of what is meant by health, and finally how nursing comes into play to help the person. These four components are all consistent with mental health nursing, which must focus on the person as a holistic individual who has both physical as well as mental health needs. General nurses have rightly been accused in the past of only seeing the physical at the expense of the psychological needs of the patient; mental health nurses should beware the reverse situation and the risk of neglecting the patient's physical health. The way a person interacts with both the physical and social environment influences their state of mental and physical health and is therefore of great concern to the fourth component of a nursing model, nursing itself. Nursing models, therefore, are built from components which are wholly consistent with mental health care.

We have also seen (p. 9) that models may be broadly grouped into one of three categories; those that are concerned with achieving a balance between systems (homeostatis), be they physical or psycho-social (systems models); those that are concerned with patient development; or those with an interactionist perspective. These three broad approaches to building nursing models are again compatible with mental health care.

Models based on systems run the danger of becoming reductionist if they only focus on physiology, and if this approach alone is used then it would be true to say this is not a suitable way forward (see p. 51 for a critique of Roper's model in this regard). However, systems and the concept of balance operate at many other levels other than cellular biology, particularly in the field of family and community (i.e. social systems) and it is in this area that many patients have problems. Systems in terms of nursing models have been described by Pearson and Vaughan (1986) as continually interacting with each other and also being susceptible to the effects of change both within and without the system, a description that applies to groups such as the family, networks of friends or employees. Viewed in this light, systems are clearly relevant to mental health.

We have already counselled caution about neglecting the person's physical health; health is a complete state of well-being that involves physical as well as psychological and social dimensions. Mental health nurses must also be prepared to promote physical health, and this needs attention to physical systems involving, for example, nutrition, elimination and cardiovascular function. Systems models have a place in mental health nursing providing they stress the importance of social systems, and also as a useful reminder to the nurse to think also about the patient's physical health. This point is illustrated further on.

A significant number of mental health problems stem from developmental difficulties involving growth and change. These processes are characterized by identifiable stages but do not necessarily flow in a smooth, constant, linear way. Progression can involve going backwards to go forwards (cyclical) or may involve a series of branching pathways leading to different goals or a spiralling in towards an eventual goal via a circuitous route. A variety of forces drive change onwards, perhaps in differing directions as the nature of the forces in a person's life change. This analysis of development, due to Chin (1980), seems appropriate for many mental health problems, while engaging in nursing care with a client itself involves development of the nurse–client role through a series of stages.

Interactionist models are based around the way people interact with others and their environment. They seek to discover the meanings that people give to experiences and events and acknowledge the

Change

uniqueness of these meanings to individuals, stressing the importance of the nurse's understanding how the patient sees things. In the interactionist view people learn meanings and values through the way they interact with others and also take upon themselves various social roles. This approach to nursing seems to offer a potentially very useful tool in the field of mental health.

Having established that the various key principles used in the construction of nursing models are at least consistent with the sorts of problems mental health nurses will encounter, it now remains to home in on some specific models.

Elsewhere in this book care planning and the models of Roper, Roy and Orem together with the FANCAP assessment scheme have been discussed in detail in a variety of clinical settings. These approaches are more suited to the general nursing field with their emphasis on physical care, a criticism particularly valid in the case of Roper. In this chapter, therefore, it is intended to introduce some other models which are more applicable to mental health, starting with that of Orlando.

Andrews (1983) considers that the importance of Orlando's work is that she was one of the first theorists to emphasize patient participation in planning care. Orlando sees the main aim of nursing as identifying and helping the patients meet their needs. Schmeiding (1986) has pointed out that the core of this model is the relationship between patient and nurse which allows problem identification and therefore the meeting of patient needs. The importance of this step is not just confined to mental health, and as has been argued elsewhere (p. 10) is of fundamental importance in all aspects of care.

A view that characterizes Orlando's work is that a patient's presenting behaviour, whatever form that may take, is a plea for help. This requires the nurse to attempt to discover the meaning to the patient of their behaviour stating that while the person's perceptions, thoughts and feelings are internal and therefore not observable, only their behaviour and speech might give clues to these internal processes. The importance of the nurse–client interaction is stressed, with the nurse seeking to fully understand the patient's perceptions and feelings through in-depth conversation and exploration. It is a fundamental understanding of the aims of professional nursing that gives this exploration its sense of direction and makes it unique to nursing, rather than merely conversation.

The failure of nurses to explore the meanings of behaviour with patients and the problems that flow from nurses assuming they know what the behaviour means have been well described by Schmeiding in a review of the research. She is also able to give a series of real anecdotes, some of which are based in mental health care, to show how problems have arisen and been resolved by using this approach.

In summarizing the model, Andrews (1983) considers it to be a valuable guide for nursing practice, though not fully developed as a model and rather narrow in scope. It is an approach to nursing that may clearly be of benefit in many situations in mental health, although it lacks a clearly defined structure for assessment and has little to say about the patient's physical needs.

Another model deserving of attention is the Neuman model, which, according to Whall (1983) may be applied to mental health settings. This is basically a systems model but can be interpreted to include social as well as physiological systems that see the goal of nursing as maintaining equilibrium within the various systems leading to the whole person being restored to health. One problem with this view is the danger of seeing equilibrium as a static rather than a dynamic state of affairs. In the same way, health can be seen as a static state of wellness or as an active state of seeking well-being and improvement, leading to self-actualization (p. 8). If this latter view of health is subscribed to, then care must be exercised in using systems models not to fossilize the client but to achieve equilibrium in a dynamic sense. The institutionalized long-stay patient may be said to have achieved a state of equilibrium, but it is a static, dependent state leaving the person unable to cope with the changing world outside.

Consider the analogy of a car parked at rest. It is in a state of equilibrium, but it is going nowhere. Now consider that same car driving along at a steady 30 mph: This is a state of equilibrium but is a dynamic state as the forces of friction balance its tendency to accelerate: the key difference is that this car is going somewhere. Note also that if the forces acting on the car get out of balance it will either grind to a halt or accelerate out of control into a crash. In using systems models we are trying to establish equilibrium so that the client neither grinds to a halt nor has a crash, but we should be aiming for a dynamic not a static equilibrium that allows the client room for growth, development and self-actualization.

After this digression into the realms of physics we must return to the Neuman systems model and mental health! This view sees humans as whole persons constantly reacting with stressors in their environment, striving to achieve health, which is seen as a state of wellness determined by physiological, psychological, sociological and developmental factors. This concept of health appears to be a static state of affairs. The stressors to which the person responds are from within the person (intrapersonal), between persons (interpersonal) and on a larger scale in society as a whole (extrapersonal).

The key to understanding the patient's problems lies in identifying these stressors and in discovering the patient's perceptions of them, and Neuman offers a semistructured assessment schedule with which to explore these issues. The goals of nursing are to allow the patient to cope with these stressors and restore equilibrium by working within one of three areas. Primary prevention involves preventing a stressor coming into contact with a person or strengthening the person's defences against that stressor to enable them better to deal with it.

This might involve teaching strategies to avoid stress-provoking situations or teaching coping strategies should they arise. Desensitization techniques to help patients with phobic states might also come under this category. Secondary prevention involves helping the patient once a problem has occurred to try to restore stability. This may be thought of as helping the client put the pieces back together, a familiar situation in mental health nursing. Tertiary prevention looks to the future and asks what lessons can be learnt to avoid a recurrence of this problem? There is great potential here for mental health nurses to make a major contribution towards the patient's health.

A different perspective on these three groups of goals is offered by Whall (1983), who, in reviewing the application of the model to psychiatric nursing, suggests that primary prevention consists of helping patients understand that life is full of problems and can be very frustrating and difficult while the secondary level consists of working through feelings. Since admission to mental hospitals is often in response to crisis, many patients are only too aware that life is full of problems; that is why they are ill and in need, sometimes desperately so, of help. Crisis intervention and stabilizing the situation often take priority after admission, with working through feelings coming later. The tertiary level is described as assisting the client in a crisis by working with available environmental supports. Whall thus sees the tertiary level in the mental health field as working with problems once they have occurred rather than a teaching and learning process to help the patient prevent future recurrence of problems, which is what Neuman suggests. Whall's analysis is therefore less applicable to a hospital situation than perhaps to others.

Neuman's views on nursing are therefore consistent with the needs of a significant number of clients with mental health problems. The danger is that it may lead to a status quo and not emphasize sufficiently the need for the client to achieve and grow in a dynamic way. It is difficult to see how this model may be applied to the situation in which a person has lost contact with reality and is therefore unable to give answers that are rational within the nurse's own frame of reference. This same comment also applies to Orlando's approach. The key question in Neuman's assessment is to ask the patient what they consider to be their main problems; an answer to the effect that the client considers there are no problems, or answers framed within a logic that has lost touch with reality, may leave the nurse wondering which way to turn next.

The third model to be reviewed here is that due to Peplau, which with its emphasis on development and growth immediately answers the criticism made of Neuman's model above, i.e. the danger of stagnation. Peplau, according to Collister (1986), focuses on the personal interaction between client and nurse and is concerned with the development of this relationship. Anxiety and communication are key ingredients in Peplau's understanding of health for the perception of any threat, which is a process that involves communication, provokes anxiety in the person. Anxiety can be a useful coping tool that allows us to mobilize resources to deal successfully with a threat; however, it can also overwhelm the person leading to anxiety states, preoccupation and a withdrawal from the real world.

The nursing interaction with the patient first involves orientation, i.e. making the client aware that help is available and beginning to discover the reasons why the person feels in need of that help. There is a danger of relapsing into the medical model at this stage, with the interaction focusing on disease labels and means of overcoming or attempting to cure a disease entity. Peplau argues that instead the focus should be on the person's situation and problems and seeing these as part of life and an opportunity for learning. In this way the person can grow and develop through their problems in a richer and fuller sense; the experience becomes a positive life event in which the person played a major role.

This phase is followed by the process of identification, in which the client begins to identify the nurse as someone who cares and who is able to help. This in turn allows the client to express their feelings although this will be influenced by the degree of dependence the client may feel upon the nurse. The stage is now set for exploiting the strength of the nurse–client relationship and the feelings and patient perceptions that have been uncovered in an attempt to resolve problems. The meanings behind events and behaviours may be explored and goals set at this phase. This problem solving phase is therefore known as the exploitation phase and leads on to the client leaving the relationship with maximum independence, the resolution phase.

Peplau's model does not offer a structured assessment tool, and as Pearson and Vaughan (1986) have observed, it would be inappropriate if it did, as the core of her model is the forming of a relationship with the client, particularly during the orientation phase. The mental health nurse uses a whole range of skills, and his or her own experience base, in exploring the patient's mental state. This approach does not lend itself to a rigidly structured assessment tool since the assessment is as much patient-led as nurse-led. It is essential, however, that written records be kept and consequently Pearson and Vaughan suggest using Maslow's hierarchy of needs and the SOAP process (see later) alongside Peplau's model as a means of planning and documenting care. The unstructured nature of the assessment could lead to important information being missed of a physical nature and, as we have already stressed the importance of not neglecting physical health, using something like Maslow's hierarchy to lend structure and remind the nurse of important physiological parameters is worthwhile. Alternatively, the FANCAP assessment scheme (p. 48) could be used here, although this is shown in use with King's model later in this chapter.

The letters in SOAP stand for Subjective experiences and feelings of the client (S), Objective observations made by the nurse such as height and weight (O), Assessing the client using subjective and objective information that has been gathered to formulate problem statements (A), and finally deciding on a Plan of action (P). We have already seen that an excellent assessment form consists of a blank piece of paper (p. 103) and such a form is ideally suited to a wide range of nursing situations including the SOAP format.

According to Reed and Johnston (1983), Peplau's model has served as a basis for psychodynamic nursing since 1952, when her early work was first published, and has remained a valid model for nursing psychotherapy ever since. It may be said that the model is limited in the number of situations in which it can be applied as it requires a great deal of one-to-one interaction and is therefore time-consuming and its use depends upon the client's ability to recognize that he or she has problems. However, we have argued elsewhere that models should be chosen to suit individual clients' needs, there can be no universal model, and it has to be said that whatever approach is followed, it is difficult to help a client who does not recognize that he or she has a problem in the first place.

Peplau's emphasis on good communication is a lesson that all nurses should take on board whatever their speciality and she should also be given credit for being one of the first nurse theorists to try and expound a model of something that is uniquely nursing-based on inductive reasoning from a great deal of observational work. Peplau even predates the leading figure of modern nursing, Virginia Henderson, and must to some extent have influenced that redoubtable lady.

Peplau's main emphasis is on the way people relate to each other and, as Collister points out, this requires the nurse to 'know thyself' as a person and also maintain a neutral non-judgemental attitude to the client throughout the interaction. The need for a high degree of self-awareness on behalf of the nurse in this model has implications for nursing education as self-awareness training needs to be included in curriculum design if Peplau's model is to be used. Nurses in the general field might also benefit from such an approach since they too have to remain emotionally neutral through some very difficult situations. The use of primary nursing will bring nurses closer to patients, which in turn means the nurse must feel more confident in himself or herself in order for relationships to develop. Primary nursing demands that nurses build relationships with patients which will parallel the phases described by Peplau; her work is therefore of great relevance to all nurses, not just those involved in mental health care.

The final model that will be briefly reviewed is that of Imogene King. She places the emphasis again on social interaction, although there are strands of systems theory present in her work. King is concerned principally with the way social systems, interpersonal relationships, perception and health are linked together through interactions between people. Problems in the field of mental health commonly arise out of interpersonal relationships and also the social setting of the individual, while the client's perceptions of reality may also lead the person into severe difficulties. Health is seen as coping with stress and being able to function within social roles. The model therefore seems relevant to mental health problems and has a view of health that should be acceptable to nurses in this field.

Interaction with other people in pursuit of common goals leads to three sets of systems, personal, interpersonal and social, and according to Aggleton and Chalmers (1990), the nurse must understand each of these systems and how they affect each other in order that high-quality care may be delivered with the King model.

The personal system is about the client's self-concept, while the interpersonal system relates to communication and interaction with others. The final system, the social system, is concerned with groupings within society which in their turn influence the individual, such as family or the health-care service itself. Notions of power and authority are inherent in this system and may be very relevant to the problems experienced by some clients.

The nurse needs to explore King's three systems with the patient in the assessment stage, seeking both objective and subjective information. This process of interaction should be geared towards arriving at a mutual, shared understanding of problems and goals as the three systems are explored. This process allows the agreement of common goals, and it is this process of mutual goal setting between nurse and patient that is fundamental to King's model. The interaction of human beings with each other and their environment which leads to goal attainment is defined by King (1986) as transaction, the fundamental goal of nursing intervention. King emphasizes the need to prevent health problems occurring as well as the need to help the client once problems have arisen, a fact that should be borne in mind during client–nurse interaction.

Various writers have made the point (e.g. Pearson and Vaughan, 1986) that communication and perception are crucial to the successful outcome of nursing care using King's model. King (1986) herself proposes that the interaction process will be influenced by the perceptions of nurse and client. Major difficulties in working towards mutually agreed goals may unfortunately arise if the client's perceptions of reality are seriously distorted. However, an appreciation of the client's perception of reality is clearly a prerequisite for nursing care and in this sense King's emphasis on this facet of nurse–client interaction is a strength. Mutual goal setting or transactions may have to be postponed until the client has a clearer perception of reality, as King herself states that perceptual accuracy is necessary in nurse–client interactions, along with an accurate perception of time and space, for transactions to occur. This of course raises the issue of what reality is, a debate that has exercised the minds of great philosophers since human beings first evolved the ability to think!

King therefore requires nurses to explore the client's world in terms of the client's self-concept, relationships with individuals and with the larger social groups and forces within society. Nursing interventions involve transactions with the client, i.e. setting goals that both parties agree will be helpful in allowing the patient to reduce stress and function within his or her various social roles. A wide range of nursing skills is necessary in this context, particularly drawn from the field of counselling. Change and development of the relationship is to be encouraged, with the client increasingly taking the lead in interactions; however, the nurse needs to ensure that transactions remain realistic.

As we saw with Peplau's model, the assessment lacks structure and it would be very easy, while concentrating on the client's personal, interpersonal and social systems, to miss important physical aspects of his or her well-being. Physical health problems may exist concurrently with mental problems and be closely linked. Examples of a few such common problems are listed below.

(1) A depressed client may, for example, have neglected eating and drinking, leading to weight loss, dehydration and a poor nutritional status, which can lead on to many other health problems.
(2) Chronic pain can lead to clients feeling low and depressed.
(3) Problems such as constipation, stress incontinence or a urinary tract infection may exert a negative effect on the way a client feels.
(4) Inactivity may be reflected in poor standards of personal hygiene and neglect.
(5) Smoking leads to many health problems of which those affecting the respiratory and cardiovascular systems are the most obvious.
(6) Frustration, anxiety, depression and feelings of worthlessness are commonly observed amongst patients in general hospital and community settings suffering from severely limited physical

In view of the key role played by communication in King's work, it is suggested that the assessment be structured around the FANCAP scheme (p. 48). The reader will recall that the 'C' stands for communication and it would be appropriate therefore to commence the assessment by exploring the patient's mental status in a general way with the aid of King's sytems under that heading, before moving on to a more structured assessment of the physically oriented headings of fluids (F), aeration (A), nutrition (N), activity (A) and pain (P).

Communication should start with the patient's personal system, looking at his or her perceptions, self-concept and body image, growth and development along with the client's views of space and time. The interpersonal system requires the nurse to discover the client's views on roles, significant others in the person's life and interactions with others. Both verbal and non-verbal communication should be assessed along with stress reactions and coping mechanisms before moving on to see how the client feels about larger-scale social systems such as relationships within the family. The route the nurse follows to explore these areas will be unique to each individual patient and should be as flexible as possible before moving into the more structured, physically orientated, assessment.

King's model has various implications for nursing, the most obvious of which is a willingness to treat the client as an equal partner in care, which marks a major divergence from some of the more traditional schools of thought. Without this concept of equality, mutual goal setting and meaningful transactions will be hampered. King emphasizes individuals' rights to have knowledge about themselves and their right to participate fully in decisions affecting their health and lives, including the right to refuse health care.

A logical step from this position is the right of the client to share access to information held about the client. It is interesting, therefore, to note the results of research by Essex *et al.* (1990) into shared care records for mentally ill patients. They studied a situation in which clients' information was recorded in non-technical language and the clients themselves were invited to make entries into the records. Of the 51 persons involved almost all said they liked to see what was written about them and being asked for their comments. GPs were also enthusiastic about the scheme, but psychiatrists involved were unhappy about the project. Community nurse managers were sadly recorded as lacking in any interest in the idea. Does this mean that the nurses in question were not prepared to accept clients as partners in care?

The use of King's model also requires nurse education to embrace communication skills as a major aspect of care while challenging traditional ideas of the nurse as in some way superior to the client. For a nurse to feel comfortable in a joint goal-setting exercise, that nurse must also feel comfortable in himself or herself. Self-awareness is a key element here, as in the work of Peplau. The education of nurses in the field of mental health already embraces communication skills and self-awareness, so their requirement as part of a curriculum based on King's model should be no barrier to such developments.

King's model, in conjunction with the FANCAP scheme, has been successfully used for teaching mental health nursing as part of undergraduate nursing studies at Bristol Polytechnic for 5 years. It clearly has great potential in a wide range of fields of mental health nursing, and Gonot (1983), after a rigorous analysis, has concluded that it has great practical value in terms of contributing to nursing research, education and clinical practice.

In briefly reviewing these four models it has become apparent that the concepts and ideas they embrace have a lot to contribute to mental health nursing, and also should give general colleagues food for thought. Key ingredients such as notions of growth and development along with respect for the individual and the effects of social and environmental factors in producing behaviour prevail. The client's view of the world and the meanings attached to those views are emphasized while the nature of interpersonal relationships is explored on many levels. There is therefore a rich framework of ideas contained within these four models alone that could form a basis for the development of mental health nursing as a profession in its own right, growing away from the traditional domination of the medical profession. Given the huge problems facing mental health care today, it might be thought a tall order to expect nurses to cope with all that and explore new ground in pursuit of excellence. It is, but do not nurses in all fields owe it to their patients as well as themselves to seek the best?

The discussion so far has suggested that there are some potentially very useful conceptual frameworks available for development in mental health. The reader is reminded of the discussion earlier in this book about the need to be flexible, adapting, maybe mixing parts of models as part of the process of development to suit particular requirements. That is equally as valid in mental health care as in any other field of nursing endeavour.

It will make an interesting conclusion to this chapter to look at a substantial piece of research into the attitudes of sisters and charge nurses in long-stay psychiatric wards towards nursing models. McKenna (1989) surveyed all staff in these grades in Northern Ireland; his final sample comprised 95 nurses out of a possible 98. He found only 5.3% had attended any meeting specifically to discuss nursing models, while only a further 27.4% had heard them mentioned in passing at meetings. Of the rest they stated that they either had had a photocopied article sent to them to display on a notice board (usually a rather ineffective means of communication) or simply admitted they knew nothing of them. The reader is reminded of Smith's plea for the professionalization of mental health nursing earlier in this chapter.

McKenna then prepared a summary of how 19 nursing models each treated the key elements of health, person, environment and nursing and asked the subjects to indicate which they supported as most suitable for their patients. He used interviews as well as this questionnaire approach to gather further information.

The validity of this research must be open to question since most of the subjects clearly had little or no knowledge about nursing models. The reliability of the responses to a matrix of 19 alternative model descriptions is questionable; further there is no mention of piloting this stage of the work. Without piloting it is possible that some respondents may have misunderstood the wording of the statements. It is also questionable how valid the researcher's model summaries were, as there is no evidence of a validation exercise. There was scope for the introduction of personal bias at this stage.

These are serious questions to be borne in mind when looking at the results. McKenna found that the overwhelming preference amongst the subjects was for the health needs model of Minshull *et al.*, then Roper and Henderson's models. Minshull *et al.* (1986) discussed a health needs model, which they admit is very simplistic, based on Maslow's hierarchy of needs. Authors such as Webb (1984) have been critical of the overuse of Maslow in nursing. Minshull's thesis that unmet needs constitute a patient problem which will be met by the nurse, by implication acting for the patient to fill those needs, is logically sound but hardly original. This is surely the language of Virginia Henderson. Minshull *et al.*, therefore, while rightly emphasizing health promotion in their work, seem to be very close to Henderson's original ideas.

There was hardly any support for the sort of models discussed in this chapter, with their focus on mental functioning, social interactions, growth and development. Does this reflect the serious problems in the design of the study outlined above or the views of the staff in these long-stay areas? If the latter is the case we have a situation where mental health nurses would prefer to use models that were developed for physical illness, some of which have been the subject of considerable criticism.

How valid are such models as a basis for care of the long-term mentally ill, except as a basis for institutional care? It may be argued that some patients in long-stay settings are not thought really capable of forming relationships or social interaction, which incidentally is all the more reason to try to achieve these goals. However, there is for most patients some little decision that the patient can make, an opinion they can state, which represents the first step towards the sort of model-based practice discussed in this chapter, if nurses are prepared to develop their care along such lines. Mental handicap nurses have made great strides with the concept of normalization as a model of care, so maybe the approaches to nursing discussed here are viable in long-term mental health settings also.

If the physically oriented, 'doing things for the patient' models are thought valid in an institutional setting, then let us be honest about this and ask how appropriate community care would be for such patients? The indications would appear to be that a very high degree of support would be necessary to sustain patients coming directly into the community from care under such a nursing philosophy. Those resources have clearly not been available in the rest of the United Kingdom, as the sorry state of many long-term patients eloquently testifies.

One final point worthy of mention concerns the lack of in-service training available to staff in the areas studied. Demographic data revealed that 70% of this group of staff were aged 40 or over. Only 8.5% had an education up to A-level standard and 2.1% had completed the Diploma in Nursing. These characteristics suggest a lack of recent educational experience for many members of staff, while their lack of information about nursing models highlights a lack of in-service education about professional nursing issues. If managers of mental health nursing are serious about quality care, in-service education covering a whole range of issues, of which nursing models is only one, must be given a high priority.

The purpose of this chapter has been to review the position of mental health nursing as a professional discipline in its own right and to briefly discuss four of the various nursing models that offer significant potential as tools to help build a body of knowledge unique to mental health nursing. It is hoped that this chapter will stimulate thought and debate of the issues involved and also show that while mental health nursing is different in some ways from general nursing, nurses in these fields can and must learn from each other as we each face a significant number of similar problems. Nursing in any situation exists for the benefit of patients and clients whose needs derive from a mixture of physical, mental and social problems. Nursing must be flexible and integrated enough to meet that challenge.

References

Aggleton P & Chalmers H (1990) King's Model. *Nursing Times,* **86**(1), 38–39.

Andrews C (1983) Ida Orlando's model of nursing. In Fitzpatrick J & Whall A (eds) *Conceptual Models of Nursing* Bowie, Maryland: Robert J Brady Co.

Chin R (1980) The utility of systems models and developmental models for practitioners. In Riehl J & Roy C (eds) *Conceptual Models for Nursing Practice.* New York: Appleton Century Crofts.

Collister B (1986) Psychiatric nursing and a developmental model. In Kershaw B & Salvage J (eds) *Models for Nursing.* London: Wiley.

Essex B *et al.* (1990) Pilot study of records of shared care for people with mental illnesses. *British Medical Journal,* **300**(6737), 1442.

Fitzpatrick J, Whall A, Johnston R & Floyd J (1982) *Nursing Models: Applications to Psychiatric Mental Health Nursing.* Bowie, Maryland: Robert J Brady Co.

Gonot P (1983) Imogene M King: A theory for nursing. In Fitzpatrick J & Whall A (eds) *Conceptual Models for Nursing.* Bowie, Maryland: Robert J Brady Co.

King I (1986) King's theory of goal attainment. In Winstead-Fry P (ed) *Case Studies in Nursing Theory.*

New York: National League for Nurses.

Mangen SP *et al.* (1983) Cost effecctiveness of community psychiatric nurse or out patients psychiatric care of neurotic patients. *Psychological Medicine,* **13**, 407–416.

McKenna HP (1989) The selection by ward managers of an appropriate nursing model for long stay psychiatric patient care. *Journal of Advanced Nursing,* **14**, 762–775.

Minshull J, Ross K & Turner J (1986) The human needs model of nursing. *Journal of Advanced Nursing,* **11**, 643–649.

Paykell ES (1982) Community psychiatric nursing for neurotic patients: A controlled study. *British Journal of Psychiatry,* **140**, 573–581.

Pearson A & Vaughan B (1986) *Nursing Models for Practice.* Oxford: Heinemann.

Rae M (1990) Relapse risk for psychiatric in-patients. *Nursing Standard,* **4**(23), 14.

Reed PG & Johnston RL (1983) Peplau's nursing model: The interpersonal process.In Fitzpatrick J & Whall A (eds) *Conceptual Models of Nursing.* Bowie, Maryland: Robert J Brady Co.

Reed PG (1987) Constructing a conceptual framework for psychosocial nursing. *Journal of Psychosocial*

Nursing, **25**(2), 24–28.

Schmeiding NJ (1986) Orlando's theory. In Winstead-Fry P (ed) *Case Studies in Nursing Theory*. New York: National League for Nursing.

Siegler M & Osmond H (1966) Models of madness. *British Journal of Psychiatry*, **112**, 1193–1203.

Smith L (1986) Issues raised by the use of nursing models in psychiatry. *Nurse Education Today*, **6**, 69–75.

Walsh M & Ford P (1989) *Nursing Rituals, Research and Rational Action*. Oxford: Heinemann.

Webb C (1984) On the eighth day God created the nursing process and nobody rested. *Senior Nurse*, **1**(33), 22–25.

Whall A (1983) The Betty Neuman health care system model. In Fitzpatrick J & Whall A (eds) *Conceptual Models of Nursing*. Bowie, Maryland: Robert J Brady Co.

Wikinson G (1988) I don't want you to see a psychiatrist. *British Medical Journal*, **297** (Nov. 5), 1144–1145.

7 NURSING MODELS IN ONCOLOGY

The word cancer continues to be one that elicits fear and dread. Rather than a word, it is perceived as a sentence that once pronounced condemns the individual concerned to a future filled with physical and mental suffering if not eventual death. The duration of the sentence is uncertain, it may be weeks, months or years and there may be remissions for 'good behaviour'. A more accurate and informed perspective is that cancer is a chronic disease, which can have acute exacerbations but which is not synonymous with suffering and death. Although in this respect cancer has much in common with other potentially fatal chronic conditions, such as chronic obstructive airways disease and diabetes, it appears to be unique in the extent to which it threatens attitudes and beliefs and challenges coping strategies. This threat extends not only to the individual concerned but also their families, friends, colleagues and all those involved in their care. As cancer now affects one in three of the population, its impact on all of us in both our personal and professional lives cannot be ignored.

Scientific and medical developments have significantly improved the chances for cure for many patients and enabled the progress of the disease to be controlled in many more. At the other end of the spectrum the whole area of palliative care has undergone a revolution with the establishment of palliative care teams, expansion of the Macmillan nursing service and growth of the hospice movement. The emphasis is now shifting towards helping those individuals who have physically healed or have responded to treatment to repair their self esteem, have adapted to a new image of themselves and generally been rehabilitated within the limits of their illness. In the words of Cassileth (1979) 'Cancer is much more than cellular dysfunction. It is an historic event; a conceptual bias; a social, economic and ethical dilemma.'

Many nurses, because of their close and sustained contact with cancer patients and their significant others, have long realized that the sociological and psychological perspectives of cancer are as important to their patient as the physical. Unfortunately, all too often it is the traditional medical model of care that predominates, with its emphasis on physiological systems and anatomical structures and its distinction between mind and body. Such a reductionist approach is illustrated by the case of a woman who had undergone a radical vulvectomy. Her surgeon was delighted with the fact that he had made a complete excision of the malignant tissue and the nurses were delighted that her wound was healing without any infection. The patient meanwhile was becoming more and more depressed and the focus of this depression was the post-operative swelling of her right leg. It transpired that she had been told of the possibility of lymphoedema and saw this early swelling as a manifestation of its inevitability. She was terrified that this would progressively limit her mobility; interfere with her ability to continue with her present job as a sales assistant, her ability to wear fashionable clothes and her long-standing hobby of Latin American dancing. In short, this particular visible side-effect of treatment was for this patient at least as great a blow to her self-image as the removal of her vulva and impairment of sexual function, which would be concealed from all but her husband.

Recently the medical establishment have become concerned that so many patients have been seeking out complementary therapies in addition to orthodox treatment. These apparently offer individuals some means of coping with the experience of cancer and its treatment. Holism is a concept that is frequently espoused by those involved in cancer care, in an attempt to move away from the conventional mechanistic approach of the medical model. The underlying principles of holism have been described as being: responding to the person as a whole in their environment; seeing the individual as a combination of mind, body and spirit; willingness to use a range of interventions including both orthodox and complementary therapies; and encouraging the patient's self-responsibility. (British Holistic Medical Association, (1987)).

It is within this context that nurses should also be seeking to critically examine their care of patients with cancer. Oncology nursing is recognized as a specialist area of practice, but nurses will encounter patients with cancer in a wide variety of health care settings and across all age groups. To support these patients through a range of physical, emotional, social, cultural and spiritual upheavals and crises, nurses need to be what Wright (1989) describes as 'questioning creative practitioners who have the essential problem-solving skills enabling them to deal with masses of complex situations in a highly volatile and unpredictable setting'.

The use of nursing models would seem to offer some frame of reference for identifying the need for and organizing the delivery of care. It is necessary, however, to be cautious before 'jumping on the models bandwagon'. McFarlane (1986) suggests the value of nursing models is that they may:

(i) serve as tools which link theory and practice;
(ii) clarify thinking about the elements of a practice situation and their relationships to each other;
(iii) help practitioners of nursing communicate with each other more meaningfully;
(iv) serve as a guide to practice, education and research.

Luker (1989) suggests that the introduction of nursing models is an implicit criticism of practice as it is and that the models divert attention away from structural and contextual factors that limit the care that nurses are able to provide. As such she claims that they offer little more than an illusion that a change for the better is on the way. Aggleton and Chalmers (1990) also acknowledge that evaluation of a particular model's usefulness may well highlight constraints within the care environment which limit the model's ability to contribute to improved care. They emphasize the need to use this evidence to support and influence the need for change, to highlight the need for further education and research and to demonstrate the need for acquisition of specialist nursing skills.

Cancer is not one disease but many and treatment may involve surgery, radiotherapy, chemotherapy or a combination of any or all of these. Nursing of patients with malignant disease presents any nurse with an enormous challenge as, in addition to knowledge of the pathological processes, the nurse has to address ethical issues such as truth telling and informed consent and be able to give appropriate information about treatments and educate patients to enable them to be self-caring on discharge or to remain at home as outpatients. Nurses must also be aware of the problems caused by treatment, especially those related to changes in body image, and sexuality. They must have the communications skills necessary to establish trusting, supportive relationships with their partients that will allow such problems to be voiced and confronted. In addition to the knowledge and skills required to give a high standard of basic nursing, care of the cancer patient may require of the nurse advanced knowledge and skills related to management of pain and symptom control, wound care, intravenous therapy and nutrition, to highlight just a few areas of specialist practice. It is unlikely with such a diversity of needs that one model will provide all the answers in oncology nursing and an eclectic approach may be a more feasible solution. Whatever model is chosen, it should be used to guide and help the nurse to give good care and not to control or restrict the care given.

In the example cited earlier in this chapter, use of Roy's model in the patient's assessment might have provided more information within the physiological mode in relation to her need for rest and activity, and within the self-concept mode about body image. This could have led the nurse to anticipate a potential maladaptive problem and take steps to pre-empt it. Similarly, a patient presenting with a husky voice as a result of a laryngeal tumour who is admitted for a laryngectomy will also be subjected to anatomical changes that will be with him for the rest of his life. Use of Henderson's model when planning care for this patient might lead the nurse who is less experienced in the care of people with head and neck cancers to concentrate not only on the patient's loss of ability to express himself by normal speech and need to adapt to breathing through a tracheostomy but to reflect on how this will affect other fundamental needs. This would include the need to select suitable clothes, to avoid changes in the environment, and to play or participate in recreation, to illustrate some of the more obvious problem areas. If the nurse is unable to identify any need, this in itself might lead the nurse to examine his or her own deficiencies in terms of nursing knowledge. Nurses who choose to implement a self-care approach to care may find that application of Orem's model highlights the need for them to develop their teaching skills or indicates the need for further education to improve these skills (e.g. ENB 998 Teaching and assessing in clinical pracitce). An example where such an approach could readily be adopted is in paediatric oncology, where with education and support parents can be helped to remain the primary care givers. As more patients are able to receive their chemotherapy or radiotherapy treatment on an outpatient basis, so their needs and problems must be assessed fully if they are to receive individualized rather than standard care. Identification of self-care deficits using Orem's self-assessment framework would seem to offer a useful way of achieving this and may also highlight the need for resources and materials such as patient information booklets and videos that could enhance the patient's ability to be independent and self-caring.

It is hoped that this introduction and the examples that follow will illustrate that the value of using models in oncology nursing can be to encourage the nurse to examine every aspect of the patient's needs, to identify whether he or she has the necessary resources and skills required to meet those needs, and ultimately to assist the patient to achieve their full health potential.

Example 1: **Roper's model**
Sally Barlow is a 26-year-old with cancer of the cervix. Four years ago she was treated with two caesium insertions and a 6-week course of radiotherapy to her pelvic area. She has been undergoing investigations as an outpatient for a suspected recurrence involving her rectum and has today been admitted to the ward with a view to her having posterior pelvic exenteration. Sally was accompanied by Dave her boyfriend but he disappeared quickly saying that he would come back later in the day. Roper *et al.*'s ALs were used as prompts during the

assessment interview and information was documented in the order in which it was obtained.

Usual routines	Patient's problem	Goal	Nursing action
MAINTAINING A SAFE ENVIRONMENT Fully independent.	(1) Hazards of surgery (P).	No post-op complications.	Explain need for pre-op preparation. Follow standard procedures including bowel preparation.
MOBILIZING Fully independent.			
COMMUNICATING Sally observed chatting to the lady in the next bed. Talks openly about proposed surgery and says she wants as much information as possible. Becomes tearful when discussing colostomy.	See elimination.		
BREATHING P 80, BP120/80, R 16. Smokes 20 per day has tried to cut down.	(2) Breathing problems post-anaesthetic (P).	Sally will stop smoking pre-operatively.	Explain why smoking increases risks of complications. Help Sally set a time to stop. Suggest alternative stress-reducing strategies. Offer support and encouragement. Reinforce breathing and effective coughing techniques.
EATING AND DRINKING Ht 5ft 5in Wt 55 kg. Well balanced diet, no special likes or dislikes.			
ELIMINATION Urinalysis N.A.D. 1–2 bowel motions a day since radiotherapy. Recently experiencing an urgent desire to defecate — usually a false alarm. Worse at night. Occasionally passes fresh blood with her motions. Low backache for several weeks.	(3) Discomfort associated with having bowels opened (A).	No discomfort.	Offer analgesia as prescribed.
Understands surgery involves removal of 'back passage', not the bladder. Says she has been told she would need to wear a bag. Doesn't know what this entails. Feels frightened.	(4) Anxiety and fear related to lack of knowledge about colostomy (A).	For Sally to be able to discuss the impact of a colostomy on her lifestyle without becoming tearful.	Refer to specialist stoma care nurse. Provide the opportunity for Sally to voice her specific fears. Provide verbal and written information for Sally. Arrange contact with ostomist of similar age if appropriate. Sally to try wearing bag filled with water. Mark suitable sites.
PERSONAL CLEANSING AND DRESSING Fully independent.			
CONTROLLING BODY TEMPERATURE T 37.1°C.			
WORKING AND PLAYING Croupier in local casino. Socializes mainly with her family.			

Usual routines	Patient's problem	Goal	Nursing action
Is saving to buy a house with Dave.			
EXPRESSING SEXUALITY Sally and Dave live together with Sally's parents. Sally and Dave have accepted that they will not have children because of Sally's previous radiotherapy. Sally used vaginal dilators and they have been able to have vaginal intercourse. Recently Sally hasn't felt like it because of all the examinations. She is very anxious about how the surgery will affect her sexual relationship with Dave as she knows part of the vagina will have to be removed.	(5) Uncertainty about ability to have vaginal intercourse post-surgery (A).	For Sally to be able to state the potential outcome of surgery and identify some positive coping strategies.	Facilitate discussion with surgeons about this topic involving Dave according to Sally's wishes. Ensure privacy for this. Explain to Sally and Dave the resources that exist to give them support and advice with sexual difficulties post surgery.
DYING Devastated that the cancer has recurred. Says 'but I feel so well'. Feels there is no option but to have the operation. 'I'm much too young to die'. Is frightened that she will have the operation and still die.	(6) Fear of surgery and death (A).	Sally will verbally express confidence in her decision to proceed with surgery.	Allow Sally time to express all her fears. Ensure medical staff fully explain options and answer all her questions. Reinforce and help Sally interpret information given. Provide information about post-op care.
SLEEPING Normally sleeps 8–9 hours — recently disturbed (see elimination). Finding it hard to get off to sleep since she found out she had a recurrence.	(7) Lack of sleep (A).	Sally will report 8 hrs sleep.	Offer night sedation. Teach relaxation techniques.

Sally's problems are related to the forthcoming surgery and are prioritized to ensure she is physically and mentally prepared for this. Problems (4), (5) and (6) are the most important. Problems (3) and (7) are related to the cancer and will be alleviated by the operation. Sally decided to proceed with surgery and problems (1) and (2) then became priorities.

Post-operatively Sally was nursed in a high-dependency unit. After 24 hours she was transferred back to the ward and a reassessment was undertaken. As a result of this a revised care plan was formulated for Sally's post-operative care.

Usual routines	Patient's problem	Goal	Nursing actions
MOBILIZING Sally is reluctant to move in bed or sit out as she is experiencing pain (see Pain assessment chart — rated 8).	(1) Pain due to surgery (A).	Sally to rate pain less than 3.	Administer analgesia via epidural infusion. Titrate prescribed dose against pain. Inform anaesthetist if not controlling pain. Substitute oral analgesia as pain diminishes. Encourage coping strategies — distraction, massage, etc.

Usual routines	Patient's problem	Goal	Nursing actions
	(2) Complications of immobility DVT chest infections, pressure sores, etc. (P).	No avoidable complication.	Assist Sally to change her position 2-hrly whilst in bed. Encourage 2-hrly deep breathing and coughing when awake. Refer to physiotherapist. Promote mobilization by use of effective analgesia.
EATING AND DRINKING Sally has a nasogastric tube; and IVI in situ. She is NBM.	(3) Dehydration (P).	Sally to have a fluid intake of 2–3 litres/24 hrs.	Monitor and care for IVI. Administer IV fluids as prescribed. Aspirate NG. tube. Maintain fluid balance record. Provide mouth care. Introduce oral fluids and diet as instructed by surgeon.
MAINTAINING A SAFE ENVIRONMENT Sally has an abdominal wound, a perineal wound and a corrugated drain.	(4) Impaired healing due to infection (P) and previous radiotherapy (A).	Wound will be healed in 16 days.	Record vital signs 4-hrly. Administer antibiotics as prescribed. Abdominal wound — check dressing — leave intact for as long as possible. Perineal wound — repad and re-dress as necessary — shorten drain daily after 3rd day post-op. Leave all sutures for at least 14 days.
ELIMINATION Catheter in situ and draining well.	(5) Risk of UTI (P).	No UTI.	Observe, measure and record urine output. Ensure Sally remains in fluid balance and has an average urine output of >35 ml/hr. Monitor temperature 4-hrly. Maintain closed drainage system. Meatal cleansing prn.
Newly formed left ileac terminal colostomy with drainable bag attached. Small amount of haemoserous fluid.	(6) Alteration in elimination habits (a).	For Sally to manage her colostomy independently in 14 days.	Check stoma for colour and evidence of retraction 4-hrly. Measure and chart drainage. Observe for passage of flatus and stool. Administer medication to solidify stool as prescribed. In conjunction with the stoma care nurse demonstrate change of appliance with full explanation. Encourage increasing level of participation. Encourage Sally to decide on an appliance system of her choice.
PERSONAL CLEANSING AND DRESSING Restricted by IVI catheter, etc.	(7) Inability to perform own hygiene needs (A).	Sally to state she is satisfied with her appearance.	Give bed bath or assisted wash until Sally is independent. Encourage Sally to wear her own clothes.

By the ninth day post surgery Sally had made very good progress and resumed independence in all of the above activities of living with the exception of elimination. Two new problems were identified.

Usual routines	Patient's problem	Goal	Nursing action
ELIMINATION Tearful and keeps asking to have the stoma bag changed as she thinks it smells. Has not as yet touched the stoma or undertaken a bag change herself.	(8) Reluctance to assume responsibility for her stoma (A).	Sally to touch and clean stoma within 24 hrs. Sally to complete a bag change in 2 days.	Support and reassure Sally. Encourage her to start participating right away in self care by removing bag, cleaning her stoma and preparing the new bag. To change bag with assistance tomorrow and with minimal supervision the day after. Discuss dietary changes that may help to reduce flatus and discuss products that can reduce odour. Discuss arrangements for coping with the stoma at home and follow up care.
EXPRESSING SEXUALITY Sally is worried about how Dave will react to the sight of her stoma. She feels her body has been disfigured and that she wants to cover it up even at night so that Dave will not be put off.	(9) Anxiety about altered body image (A).	Sally to feel confident enough to sleep in the nude.	Encourage Sally to show Dave the stoma before discharge. Suggest interim coping strategies, e.g. wearing bag covers or a waist slip, etc.
	(10) Alteration in sexual behaviour (P).	Sally to report a satisfying sexual relationship (long term).	Get Sally's surgeon to explain what potential for vaginal intercourse exists. Identify potential problems with Dave and Sally and suggest alternative ways of love-making until heal is complete. Offer follow-up support and advice. Discuss reconstructive surgery if appropriate.

Example 2: **Orem's model**

Jim Davies is a 39-year-old man who has been admitted with non-Hodgkins lymphoma presenting with lung involvement. This diagnosis has just been confirmed following several weeks of uncertainty and numerous investigations. It is planned to give Jim his first course of chemotherapy on this admission and it is expected that he will receive further courses every 4 weeks for the next 6 months. The exact drugs he is to receive are not specified as the agents used may vary. It is important that the nurse is familiar with the potential side-effects of the specific drugs used. Some side-effects related to drugs commonly used are indicated but the reader should refer to an oncology or pharmacology text for more detail. Some of the side-effects of the therapy may only affect Jim after he has been discharged. For this reason it seems appropriate to use Orem's framework as the basis for planning his nursing care.

Normal self-care abilities	Current self care abilities
AIR	
No breathing problems until 3 months ago when Jim started to get progressively short of breath and	Respirations 21. Breathing not laboured and no pain reported. Still has dry irritating cough at times.

Normal self-care abilities	*Current self care abilities*
developed a dry unproductive cough. Breathing got worse and two weeks ago Jim had 'fluid drained from my lungs'.	

WATER

Drinks a variety of fluids — usually has 7–10 cups of tea/coffee/milk a day. Used to like to drink 5–6 pints of beer in his local on a Saturday night.	Found even small amounts of alcohol started to make him feel ill, so hasn't been to the pub for several weeks.

NUTRITION

Ht 5ft 10in Wt 72 kg. Eats a well balanced diet; wife does all the cooking but is 'health conscious'. Tends to eat two meals a day — no breakfast.	Has been 'off food' and has lost 4–5 kg in the last 3 months.

ELIMINATION

Bowels very regular every day after first cup of coffee. No problems passing urine.	Bowels have been irregular of late but not constipated. Jim puts it down to eating less.

ACTIVITY AND REST

Jim describes himself as an active man. Works as a foreman at a local factory and plays football for the works team. Says he was always on the go. Usually sleeps about 7 hours at night never in the day.	Feeling tired and listless and had to slow right up when his breathing got bad. Better now but still has little energy. Sleep has been disturbed by night sweats.

SOLITUDE/SOCIALIZATION

Married to Susan for 13 years; they have 2 children, Paul 12 and Sian 9. Enjoys an active social life and 'never had a moment to myself'.	Finds people are avoiding him and don't seem to know what to say. Feels he has to keep cheerful for Susan and the kids.

HAZARDS

Used to smoke but gave up 5 years ago. Drank regularly in his youth but cut down when he met Susan.	Has heard that chemotherapy makes hair fall out and makes people very sick and would like to know if this is true. Thinks the treatment might be worse than the disease.

BEING NORMAL

Felt life was going well and says he was just an ordinary chap, lucky to have a good job, happy marriage and lovely kids.	Feels life has become a nightmare — nothing is the same any more.

DEVELOPMENTAL

Doesn't like asking others for help, has always been very independent. Feels his wife and children have always been able to depend on him.	Is afraid of 'letting the family down'. Scared of being an invalid and of death.

HEALTH DEVIANCY

Always considered himself healthy and never took a day off sick until now. No personal experience of anyone with cancer, has only heard of people who have died.	Feels his body is out of control. Knows his diagnosis but has never heard of this sort of cancer. Has been told he will need at least 6 months chemotherapy to treat this. Jim says he wants to believe it will cure him but he is worried that the treatment is experimental and that he is just a guinea-pig.

From this assessment, Jim's self-care deficits (patient problems) are identified and prioritized to produce the following care plan. It is anticipated that care given during his initial admission and whilst having intravenous therapy will be partially compensatory, but as treatment progresses care will become more supportive-educative unless his disease should fail to respond to treatment. Although Jim's self-care deficits will need review on each admission for chemotherapy and new ones may be identified, it is likely that this care plan will also be relevant for each subsequent course of chemotherapy.

Self-care deficit	Goal	Nursing actions
(1) Inadequate knowledge of cancer in general and lymphoma in particular (A).	Jim will be able to discuss his condition knowledgeably and ask relevant questions.	Explain the nature of cancer and give verbal and written information about lymphomas and the treatment options. Encourage questions and answer as honestly as possible. Involve Susan in discussions whenever possible.
(2) Inaccurate knowledge of chemotherapy (A).	Understanding of chemotherapy demonstrated by:	Explain how chemotherapy works and the major side-effects of Jim's treatment.
	(1) Jim's ability to identify potential side-effects.	Explain how these are prevented or controlled, answering all questions as honestly as possible. Reinforce with written information that Jim can show to his family.
	(2) Jim's ability to describe his treatment plan.	Ensure Jim is kept informed of treatment plans, e.g. when chemotherapy is to be given. Reinforce information given by medical staff using terms Jim can understand. Ensure Jim knows who to contact if he has questions or problems at home.
(3) Infertility (P).	Retention of potential for future paternity.	Discuss risk of infertility with Jim and Susan and offer opportunity for sperm banking.
(4) Anorexia (A).	No further weight loss.	Explain chemotherapy may exacerbate this problem. Arrange for dietician to see Jim and Susan. Offer Jim food supplements in addition or in place of hospital food. Administer anti-emetics as required. Monitor weight on each admission.
(5) Constipation (P).	Daily motion. Soft formed stool.	Discuss dietary and fluid intake. Encourage high-fibre diet as tolerated.
(6) Weakness and lethargy (A).	Jim reports having more energy.	Reassure Jim that the treatment should not make this worse and that as the cancer responds to the drugs he should start feeling more energetic.
(7) Lack of sleep (A).	Jim reports undisturbed sleep.	Reassure Jim that night sweats are a symptom of the cancer which should disappear as treatment takes effect. Ensure Jim has changes of nightwear and bedclothes. Assist Jim with washing when they occur.
(8) Difficulty accepting the reality of his condition and adjusting to 'sick role' (A).	Jim to verablize strategies for making changes in his life during chemotherapy treatment.	Encourage discussion about potential changes Jim will need to make. Offer support for positive change

Self-care deficit	Goal	Nursing actions
		and suggestions for self-care. Encourage Jim's involvement in decisions, e.g. about time of treatment, etc. Encourage Jim to accept support from others during his treatment.
(9) Anxiety about job and loss of earnings (A).	Short term — Jim and Susan to discuss changes in family budget. Long term — Jim to return to work.	Reassure Jim that many patients return to work during treatment. Suggest he contact company personnel officer to discuss arrangements. Refer to social worker if Jim agreeable.
(10) Feels isolated from friends and family (A).	Jim to report improved communication between him and family and friends.	Encourage and provide opportunities for Jim to express his feelings. Facilitate communication between Jim and Susan by giving them information together and offering them privacy for discussion. Suggest strategies that Jim could use to make contact with friends and overcome the 'barrier' of his diagnosis.
(11) Requires intravenous injection of cytotoxic drugs.	Safe administration.	Follow hospital policy and procedures for administration of IV cytotoxic drugs.
(12) Nausea and vomiting (P).	No vomiting.	Administer anti-emetics, steroids and sedatives prior to chemotherapy and as prescribed. Evaluate effect and notify medical staff if ineffective. Provide clean vomit bowls, tissues and mouth wash as precaution and as required. Give diet as tolerated. Ensure oral medication available on discharge. Teach distraction/relaxation techniques.
(13) Poor fluid intake (P).	Fluid intake of 3 litres in 24 hrs.	Explain need for high intake in order to promote rapid excretion of drugs and metabolites. Monitor and care for IVI until hydration regime complete and Jim is able to tolerate oral fluids. Give anti-emetics.
(14) Bone marrow depression (P).	Jim will experience minimal neutropenia, anaemia, thrombocytopenia and their sequelae.	Ensure Jim and family are aware of manifestations of BMD, i.e. fevers, malaise and bleeding and bruising. Encourage good oral hygiene — need to avoid people with known infections; need to use soft toothbrush and avoid wet shave, etc. Encourage rest and conservation of energy. Explain procedures for checking blood counts and delaying treatment if count too low. Ensure Jim knows who to contact if concerned.

Self-care deficit	Goal	Nursing actions
(15) Specific side-effects of drugs used (P).	No unexpected side-effects.	Inform Jim of these and appropriate strategy for prevention.

Example 3: **Roy's model**

Mary Carter is a 44-year-old woman who has been admitted to the ward for breast surgery. She works as a midwife at a hospital some distance away and arrived unaccompanied. Mary had been attending the hospital as an out patient for 6 years because of a history of nodular breasts and a family history of breast cancer. Mammography 12 months ago was negative but when repeated 12 days ago had shown suspicious features. Needle aspiration cytology performed at the same time also indicated the presence of malignant cells. Mary had been clerked by the surgical houseman at a pre-admissions clinic and routine blood tests and a chest X-ray had been taken. Mary had also met the nurse specialist for breast care and discussed the options for surgery. A bone scan and a liver scan were also performed to establish the presence of any disseminated disease. Mary was fully aware of her diagnosis and the intended surgical procedure, which for her was a left mastectomy. The following assessment for Mary was completed using Roy's framework.

First-level assessment	Second-level assessment
PHYSIOLOGICAL MODE *Oxygenation and circulation* RR 18, BP 130/85, P82. No shortness of breath. Non-smoker. Tortuous dilated veins both legs. Causing aching legs at the end of the day.	 Varicose veins (F). Familial problem (C). Overweight (C). On her feet for long periods at work (C).
Nutrition Ht 5ft 5in Wt 75 kg increasing over last year. Looks overweight and says she finds it hard to diet. Likes dairy produce. Cooks for her father who eats very little and says she often 'finishes things off' rather than waste them.	Inappropriate diet (F). Enjoys food (C). Limited exercise (C). Unaware of association between high-fat diet and breast cancer (C). Belief that it is wrong to waste food (R).
Elimination Bowels opened daily no current difficulties. Urinary — no difficulties. Urinalysis NAD.	
Activity and rest Goes to bed about 10.30 p.m. and describes herself as a lark. No current sleeping difficulty. Enjoys swimming when she has time.	
Skin integrity Skin intact — first noticed left nipple was inverted 6 weeks ago.	Malignant lump in left breast (F). Nodular breast for many years (C). Practised BSE (C). Negative mammography 12 months ago (C). No pregnancies (C). Mother died of breast cancer (R).

First-level assessment	*Second-level assessment*

Regulation

Appears well hydrated.
Temperature 37.1°C.
Periods regular 5/28 days. LMP last week.
Gets severe premenstrual breast tenderness and increased nodularity. Often feels tense and irritable 'before the curse'.

Premenstrual syndrome (F).
Usual pattern of menses (C).
Possible hormonal imbalance (C).
Homeopathic medication (C).
Cultural beliefs about female role (R).

SELF-CONCEPT MODE

Physical

Doesn't mind losing a breast if it is the best way to ensure the cancer has all been removed. Does not want to have radiotherapy as she remembers what it did to her mother.
Says she can cope with the physical disfigurement herself but says 'no man will want me now with only one breast'.

Impending mastectomy (F).
Fears radiotherapy (C).
Memories of her mother's reactions to radiotherapy (R).
Prospect of changed body image (F).
Has seen mastectomy scars (C).
No current partner (C).
Fear of being sexually unattractive (C).
Belief about importance of breasts to men (R).

Personal

Fully aware of diagnosis and its implications. Feels angry with herself and with doctors. She believed that screening would be reliable and that she has been let down.
Thinks she should have been more assertive and asked for an earlier appointment when she first noticed a change.

Breast cancer (F).
Different feeling lump for about 3 months (C).
Negative mammography last year (C).
GP unsympathetic (C).
Known greater risk of breast cancer (C).

ROLE FUNCTION

Unmarried.
One older brother.
Cares for elderly and demanding father who has been admitted to the local cottage hospital for the duration of Mary's admission. Mary is tearful when she talks of her father and admits to feeling guilty for resenting the demands he puts on her.
RGN and SCM
Is worried at being off sick and the extra work others will have to do.

Hospitalization (F).
No support services involved in father's care (C).
Conflict between brother's wife and her father (C).
Assumption of her mother's role (R).
Demanding job (F).
Expectations of self (C).

INTERDEPENDENCE

Has always thought of herself as very independent. Finds it hard to ask for help. Feels she should be able to cope with the surgery because she is a nurse and 'knows what it is all about'. Doesn't want to be a nuisance or treated differently because of being a nurse. Says there are many people much worse off than her.

Hospitalization (F).
Familiarity with hospital staff and routines (C).
First time she has been a patient (C).
Breast cancer (F).
Normally self-reliant (C).
Perception that nurses are 'difficult patients' (R).

From this assessment the following maladaptive problems were identified:

(1) Potential risk of DVT or pulmonary embolism.
(2) Excessive weight gain.
(3) Inverted L. nipple.
(4) Anxiety about (i) spread of cancer, (ii) radiotherapy.
(5) Feelings of loss related to potential altered body image.
(6) Anger that preventive actions have not been effective.
(7) Guilt about inability to continue caring for her father.

(8) Conflict between professional role and sick role.
(9) Difficulty accepting dependence on others.

Problem (3) will be addressed by surgery and problem (1) will be important in the post-operative period. Problem (2) is a long-term problem and does not have priority at this stage. All the remaining problems will be relevant throughout Mary's admission and the following care plan was devised pre-operatively.

Problem	Goal	Nursing actions
Hazards of surgery (P).	No avoidable complications.	Follow standard pre-op preparation following hospital policy.
Anxiety (A).	Mary will say (a) she is more confident the cancer has not spread, (b) she is less frightened of radiotherapy.	Encourage Mary to express her fears. Discuss route of spread and remind Mary negative scans. Provide written information on sources of support, e.g. Mastectomy Association. Reassure Mary of follow-up care. Provide written and verbal information about radiotherapy. Introduce her to a patient who has recently had radiotherapy.
Anger (A).	Mary to say she feels less angry.	Encourage Mary to express her feelings by writing them down and asking the doctors to explain why the tests were negative. Teach stress-reduction techniques and encourage Mary to identify ways she could be more assertive in the future.
Difficulty accepting dependence on others (A).	Mary to accept her need for temporary dependence.	Identify Mary's previous coping mechanisms. Encourage Mary to identify her support network and to identify who might be of most help to her at this time. Identify gaps in Mary's informal support system and suggest what 'formal' help might be available.
Difficulty accepting transition from nurse to patient (A).	Mary to temporarily relinquish her 'nurse role'.	Encourage Mary to verbalize her feelings about being a patient. Establish her knowledge base prior to giving information to ensure it is pitched at an appropriate level. Encourage Mary to ask questions and facilitate her participation in decision making. Ensure nursing staff give Mary the same amount of attention as other patients while respecting her professional status.

Following surgery and Mary's return to the ward her condition was reassessed and her care plan was revised.

First-level assessment	Second-level assessment
PHYSIOLOGICAL MODE *Oxygenation and circulation* RR 15, BP 110/75, P74.	Narcotic analgesia (F).

First-level assessment	Second-level assessment
Nutrition and fluids NBM for over 8 hrs. IVI	Anaesthetic (F). Pre-op fasting (C).
Elimination Last passed urine pre-operatively.	Anaesthetic (F). Pre-op fasting (C).
Activity and rest Drowsy but can move left arm when asked.	Surgery (F). Left breast cancer (C).
Skin integrity Left Patey mastectomy scar covered in Op-Site dressing. Two Redivac drains, one to mastectomy flap and one to axilla.	As above.
Regulation IVI.	Surgery (F). NBM (C).
Temperature 36.3°C.	Anaesthetic (F). Cold operating theatre (C).
IM Omnopon and Fentazin given in recovery. Mary says she has very slight discomfort; 2 on a scale of 1–10.	Pain (F). Surgery (C).
SELF-CONCEPT MODE Asking if all the cancer has been removed.	As above.
ROLE FUNCTION Asking if her brother has telephoned.	As above. Next of kin (C).
INTERDEPENDENCE Inability to fulfil all physical needs.	Surgery (F). IVI, Redivac drains, etc. (C).

Care plan problem	Goal	Nursing action
Hypovolaemic shock (P).	Systolic BP will remain above 100.	Monitor vital signs ½–4/hrly. Observe wound and drains for excessive blood loss.
Inability to use L. arm due to pain (A).	Short term — Mary will say she has no pain.	Administer analgesia within prescribed limits taking account of vital signs. Evaluate using pain scale and report to medical staff if analgesia not effective. If pain is well controlled, commence oral medication once Mary is eating and drinking.
	Long-term — Mary will be able to raise her arm to shoulder level within 5 days and will have regained full range of movement in 4 weeks.	Refer to physiotherapist for instruction on exercises. Reinforce teaching and encourage regular exercises. Advise Mary prior to discharge about beneficial and harmful activities. Encourage Mary to resume swimming.

135

Care plan problem	Goal	Nursing action
Insufficient fluid intake (P).	Mary will have a fluid intake of 2.5 litres in the first 24 hrs.	Maintain and monitor IVI until Mary tolerates oral fluids. Check Mary does not require a blood transfusion before removing cannula.
Risk of DVT or pulmonary embolus (P).	No DVT or PE.	TED stockings until mobile. Encourage leg exercises when awake until mobile. Encourage Mary to be fully mobile within 24 hours.
Nausea and vomiting (P).	No nausea or vomiting.	Provide vomit bowl, tissues and mouthwash, etc. Administer anti-emetics as required and evaluate effect. Commence oral fluids when awake and increase as tolerated.
Oedematous left arm (P).	Short-term — no post-op oedema.	Elevate arm on 1–2 pillows. Ensure left arm is not used for BP measurement, IVI or blood sampling.
Retention of urine (P).	Mary to pass urine within 12 hours.	Maintain IVI and encourage fluids when awake. Offer commode rather than bed pan to promote normal micturition. Note time Mary passes urine and volume.
Impaired healing due to infection or fluid collection (P).	Wound will heal without infection or fluid collection.	Monitor temperature 4-hrly. Observe wound for oozing of blood or serous fluid. Leave Op-Site intact for as long as possible. Check wound drains hourly for 24 hrs then 4-hrly for patentcy, vacuum and amount and type of drainage. Remove when drainage is less than 25 ml. in 24 hrs. Observe mastectomy flaps for any fluid collection. Remove sutures as instructed by surgeon.
Impaired thermoregulation (P).	Mary's temperature to be back to 37.1°C within 4 hours.	Provide extra blankets or use space blanket to insulate Mary from further heat loss.
Arm lymphoedema due to surgery, trauma or infection (P).	Mary will not develop arm lymphoedema.	Explain potential risks realistically without provoking unnecessary anxiety. Give advice on hand and arm care and reinforce with written information. Assess factors in Mary's life that might cause trauma to her arm e.g. gardening or needlework, etc.

Care plan problem	Goal	Nursing action
		Suggest strategies for avoiding trauma, e.g. gloves or using thimble, etc.
Anxiety about spread of disease (A).	Mary will start to identify coping strategies to enable her to manage this.	When Mary is fully conscious, get surgeon to explain the surgery that he performed. Explain it will take some days to get pathology result. Encourage Mary to verablize her anxieties about further treatment, etc. Explain how Mary's follow-up will be arranged. Encourage Mary to make plans for her future.
Change in body image (A).	Mary will look at and touch her scar; will select an appropriate bra and demonstrate her ability to fit a temporary prosthesis prior to discharge.	Be with Mary when she looks at herself in the mirror for the first time, and encourage her to express how she feels. Get Mary to wear her bra with a temporary prosthesis once the drains have been removed. Encourage Mary to wear her own clothes in the ward. Show Mary different types of prosthesis available and provide her with relevant literature on prostheses and clothing. Arrange follow-up with specialist nurse for fitting with bra and swimming costume. Discuss opportunities for future breast reconstruction. Tell Mary about support groups and give her their literature.
Feeling of guilt about her father (A).	For Mary to accept her need for support as her father's carer.	Co-ordinate meeting between Mary, her brother and the social worker to discuss her father's needs.
Overweight (A).	Mary to lose 2 kg by discharge and 1 kg per week for 6 weeks.	Discuss relationships between high-fat diet and breast cancer. Refer to dietitian.

Discussion

The Roper, Logan and Tierney (1985) model of nursing is familiar to many British nurses as it has been adopted as a framework giving structure to the curriculum of many schools of nursing and has been implemented in a wide variety of clinical areas. It is essentially a British interpretation of Henderson's ideas concerning the need of all individuals to perform certain fundamental activities of daily living (ADLs). Like Henderson's 14 ADLs, Roper *et al.*'s 12 activities of living (ALs) can be separated into those with a biological basis and those which, while integral to living, are non-essential, being concerned more with the quality of life. In this respect it would appear to address issues of fundamental importance to nurses caring for patients with cancer, e.g. the expression of sexuality and also specifically the subject of dying.

Its application to Sally's care illustrates some of the strengths and problems of using this model in practice. On admission, Sally was essentially independent in most of the ALs, and this is a feature common to many patients facing the prospect of radical treatment for cancer. The planned surgery had enormous implications for Sally in terms of potential alteration in the AL of eliminating and in her ability to express sexuality in the conventional way. Thus, the focus of Sally's care both pre-operatively, post-operatively and in the long term was the physical and psychological difficulties experienced in relation to these two ALs, while physical aspects of care related to survival and safety were the priorities of care in the immediate pre- and post-operative period.

Sally's problems that have a physical or biological basis were readily identified using the model and 'scientific knowledge' could be applied to resolve them, e.g. in relation to wound care or catheter care. It is less easy to apply the model when problems have a social or behavioural foundation, because Roper *et al.* address these aspects only superficially. In this example, Sally finds her stoma offensive. We can provide her with better appliances or air fresheners but we are not specifically encouraged to explore her socio-cultural beliefs about elimination, environmental factors such as toilet facilities at home and at work, or how Sally can be helped to return to her previous job and disguise a colostomy bag or the gurgling noises her stoma makes beneath flimsy evening wear. With experience, the nurse would anticipate these potential problems and would explore the wider social context in which Sally lives and works. It would then have to be decided whether these problems were still related to elimination or whether they would be more appropriately considered under the ALs personal cleansing and dressing and working and playing.

This highlights one of the practical difficulties commonly experienced with this model, that the interrelationship of many of the ALs makes it difficult to decide where to locate information. Sally was tearful when discussing her colostomy — this is part of non-verbal communication, but should this behaviour be recorded under communicating or eliminating?

Finally, in considering Sally's case there is the problem of defining the goals, especially in relation to problems that are related to fear and anxiety. Roper *et al.* state that goals should not be imposed and should wherever possible be expressed as behaviour that can be observed or measured. It may be that, after helping Sally review all the relevant information, her decision is not to proceed with surgery at all. In her role as patient advocate the nurse must support Sally in this decision with all its implications, even though the outcome is not the goal originally agreed.

Pain has been highlighted as an area of difficulty when implementing the Roper *et al.* model. It was not identified as such in Sally's case but should be considered if it is intended to use the model for other patients. Pain is not a primary focus for assessment in this model and is discussed under the biological aspects of living with superficial mention of its psychogenic components. These are of great importance when considering the chronic nature of much cancer-related pain. The authors' solution to this difficulty is to suggest that unless the pain interferes with a specific AL it should be documented under communication. The justification for this is that the perception of pain requires an intact nervous system. In reality this suggests that the model retains a mainly mechanistic approach, which could cause the nurse to neglect the psychological cause of the distress or fail to identify pain as an indirect cause of problems in any of the other ALs.

Orem's model of care focuses on the role of the nurse in assisting individuals to meet their own self-care requirements (Orem, 1985). Inherent in this approach is the belief that patients participate in the decision-making process about the management of their illness and the circumstances surrounding their quality of life. This may only be achieved if patients are in possession of the facts concerning their diagnosis and prognosis. The nurse–patient relationship is perceived as being complementary. Nurses act to help patients achieve responsibility for their health-related self-care by making up for deficiencies in capabilities for self-care; by supplying the necessary conditions for patients to withhold self-care for therapeutic reasons, or by maintaining, increasing or restoring self-care capabilities in order to promote independence. This can be achieved by a variety of methods such as acting for, teaching, guiding and supporting the patient, and providing the right environment for growth and development of the patient. For nurses caring for patients with cancer, characterized by its chronic course and often intermittent contact with the health care system, this model has much to commend it.

Some of the criticisms of Orem's model that are relevant to oncology are considered before discussing its usefulness in guiding care in Jim's case. Pain is an issue poorly addressed by Orem because it is only described as a contributory cause of self-care deficits. The onus is on the nurse to identify its contribution to either physical or psychological problems in any of the universal, developmental, or health-deviation self-care requisites. Walker and Campbell (1989) point out that pain does not appear in the index of Orem's work and suggest that failure to emphasize its importance in the assessment scheme is detrimental to the concept of holistic care. Conflicts and inconsistency in the model are also apparent when considering care of terminally ill and dying patients. Orem states that the aim of care in such situations is to enable patients to live as themselves, understand their illness, to approach death in their own particular way. If the patient and/or his or her family choose to use denial as their coping mechanism, the nurse may go along with this but would then fail to assist the patient and family to understand the projected outcome of the disease or prepare for the future.

Other difficulties arise when patients are unable to comply with medically defined treatments. Take, for example, the case of a single mother with ovarian cancer who is experiencing difficulty with child care during her hospitalization for monthly chemotherapy. The mother is admitted for her treatment but is told that she needs a blood transfusion first that would delay treatment for at least 24 hours. The partient at this point wishes to discharge herself because there is no one to care for her daughter. Thus, the patient's social circumstances and the patient's own role as dependent care agent for her daughter take priority over the patient's own universal self-care requisites; care must be adapted accordingly.

In Jim's case, use of Orem's model usefully highlighted his need for knowledge and support and guidance in maintaining the ability to be self-caring throughout his chemotherapy treatment. Nurses acted for Jim during the actual administration of the treatment and provided an environment which on subsequent admissions could enable Jim to make decisions about the timing of his treatment, and the management of his symptoms, enabling him to achieve minimum disruption to his family life. Such a model could apply equally well to a patient undergoing radiotherapy.

While there is no specific assessment category that is concerned with issues related to sexuality and body image, the more objective aspects of the effects of cancer and its treatment on the individual would be considered under 'being normal' rather than under 'health deviancy', which would be concerned with the more subjective.

Roy's model considers the person to be a bio-psycho-social being in constant interaction with an ever-changing environment (Roy, 1984). She identifies the recipients of nursing care as being people who have problems coping with their internal or external environment manifested by maladaptive behaviour in one of four modes, the physiological mode being concerned with structure and function; the self-concept mode with psychological needs, mental function and feelings; the interdependence mode with the need for social integrity and relationships with others; and the role function mode with psycho-social integration and expectations of society. The individual's level of or maladaption within each mode is determined by a combination of focal, contextual and residual stimuli, and the nurse's role is to promote adaptation by manipulating the stimuli appropriately. This is assumed to conserve energy, making it available for investment in the healing process and responding to new stimuli.

This model has been used successfully in the care of dying people. Behaviours that are considered ineffective in other situations, e.g. fear, denial, anger, depression, are considered to be adaptive during death, and the model also emphasizes that the recipient of care may include the individual family or groups. Chadderton (1986) and Logan (1988) have both explained their use of this model to effectively guide care given in palliative care and hospice settings. A further advantage of this model is for the care of the patient with cancer-induced pain, as the issue of pain is specifically assessed under the regulatory processes in relation to sensory experience. Walker and Campbell (1989) suggest that Roy's model has all the elements required to make a comprehensive assessment of pain in terms of manifestation, causes, influences and consequences.

In applying Roy's model when planning Mary's care, assessment of adaptation in the physiological mode was based on the five basic needs described in Roy (1984) which includes skin integrity. This was felt to be an important need area in Mary's case as she was to undergo surgery which would disrupt the skin but also because of her anxieties related to her fear of radiotherapy and its disfiguring effect on the skin, which she remembered from her mother's treatment.

Webb (1986) and Gerrish (1989) have both commented on the difficulties experienced in separating behaviours into specific modes, and this problem was experienced when writing Mary's assessment. Was Mary's weight problem related to nutrition or to self-copcept, and was her difficulty making the transfer between the role of nurse to one of patient related to role function or interdependence? It was also difficult deciding whether to classify Mary's acceptance of a mastectomy as representing adaptive behaviour in coming to terms with the potential loss of her breast, or whether it was maladaptive and indicative of low self-esteem or maladaptive because it indicated an insufficient knowledge about current methods of radiotherapy. Roy leaves adaptation undefined and this leads to problems being identified on the basis of value judgements by the nurse, unless the nurse makes strenuous attempts to validate the patient's own views of the situation.

One advantage that makes Roy's model an attractive one to use with cancer patients is the relatively equal focus it places on physiological, psychological and social needs. However, it can take considerable experience and confidence to utilize the assessment framework and, although experienced oncology nurses may find it easy to recognize and classify maladaptive behaviours within the four modes and identify the relevant stimuli in practice, the less experienced nurse may have difficulty with this.

In this chapter, three models have been applied to the care of patients with cancer. Each has been demonstrated to offer certain advantages both in theory and in practice. All three have some inherent difficulties which become apparent in actual usage and it becomes obvious that in some situations and for some patients one model could be more useful in guiding practice than another. The advantage of all the models, and others not considered here, is that they are themselves a stimulus, encouraging the nurse to reflect on more than the physical aspects of care. The nurse with expertise in oncology may already achieve this, but it is suggested that nurses caring for cancer patients in non-specialized settings may find a model-based approach invaluable in reassuring themselves that they have attempted to give their patients 'holistic' care.

References

Aggleton P & Chalmers H (1990) Model future. *Nursing Times,* **86** (3), 41–43.

British Holistic Medical Association (1987). In *Lampada Spring (II),* p. 46. London: Royal College of Nursing.

Cassileth BR (1979) *The Cancer Patient: Social and Medical Aspects of Care.* Lea and Febiger.

Chadderton H (1986) A stress adaptation model in terminal care. In Kershaw B & Salvage J (eds). *Models for Nursing.* Chichester: Wiley.

Fitzpatrick J & Whall A (1983) *Conceptual Models of Nursing; Analysis and Application.* Bowie, Maryland: Robert J Brady Co.

Gerrish C (1989) From theory to practice. *Nursing Times,* **85** (35), 42–45.

Logan M (1988) Care of the terminally ill includes the family. *The Canadian Nurse,* **84** (5), 30–34.

Luker K (1989) This house believes that nursing models provide a useful tool in the management of patient care. In Pritchard AP (ed) *Cancer Nursing. A Revolution in Care.* London: Macmillan.

McFarlane J (1986) The value of models for care. In Kershaw B & Salvage J (eds) *Models for Nursing.* Chichester: Wiley.

Orem DE (1985) *Nursing. Concepts of Practice.* New York: McGraw-Hill.

Rambo BJ (1984). *Adaptation Nursing: Assessment and Intervention.* Philadelphia: W.B. Saunders.

Roper N, Logan WW & Tierney AJ (1985) *The Elements of Nursing,* 2nd edn. Edinburgh: Churchill Livingstone.

Roy C (1984) *Introduction to Nursing: An Adaptation Model,* 2nd edn. Englewood Cliffs: Prentice-Hall.

Walker JM & Campbell SM (1989) Pain assessment, nursing models and the nursing process. In Akinsanya JA (ed) *Recent Advances in Nursing 24: Theories and Models of Nursing.* Edinburgh: Churchill Livingstone.

Webb C (1986). *Women's Health: Midwifery and Gynaecological Nursing.* London: Hodder and Stoughton.

Wright S (1989) This house believes that nursing models provide a useful tool in the management of patient care. In Pritchard AP (ed) *Cancer Nursing. A Revolution in Care.* London: Macmillan.

This book has attempted to explore some of the practical issues surrounding care planning and the use of nursing models. It remains to conclude by looking to the future and seeing how some of the major issues facing nursing today relate to the issue of nursing models.

The reform of nursing education and nursing models

The long-overdue reform of nursing education is proceding at a much slower rate than most educationalists would like because of government underfunding. Whatever the speed, it is clear that if new curricula are being designed to reflect a new approach to nursing, then nursing models should be an integral part of such changes.

Project 2000 aims to shift the emphasis away from the traditional medical model, which tends to see human beings as pieces of malfunctioning anatomy and physiology. This reductionist approach fails to see the patient as an integrated whole human being with a psychological and a social dimension as well as the physiological, or with a health and wellness dimension as well as disease and illness. This traditional view reflects the way nursing has developed in its subservient role to medicine. Project 2000 also aims to produce a nurse who can practise just as readily in the community as in hospital.

If Project 2000 is to produce a new type of nurse, a nurse who sees the patient as a holistic human being and who recognizes the importance of positive health promotion, then a new approach to nursing is required. Most models of nursing are constructed around an integrated view of a human being interacting with the environment to produce a state of health. Nursing is then sited within this framework and described in terms that reflect the author's views of how health, human beings and their social and physical environment react together. This is the approach required for nursing if we are to be true to the principles of Project 2000, anything less would merely be paying lip service.

143

At this point, reference should be made to the criticisms of Pender (1984), who has suggested that many nursing models fail to pay due attention to health promotion. Pender (1987) further considered that health promotion was a dynamic process directed towards growth and improvement in well being; she also saw it as intrinsically different from disease prevention. Detailed analysis by Hartweg (1990), comparing the work of Pender and others (notably Brubaker, 1983) with Orem's work, has demonstrated that these concepts are consistent and that health promotion is readily seen as self-care activity. Dunn (1990) has confirmed the value of the Orem model in health education by showing how it is used for health promotion in alcohol-dependent patients.

Such rigorous analysis is needed for all models of nursing if they are to be considered appropriate components of Project 2000 education. Roy's ideas, for example, of patients actively striving to adapt to stressors in their environment, implies a dynamic process (Rambo, 1984) but also suggests a reactive rather than a proactive view of the person. However, successful adaptation can be seen as an essential prerequisite for growth and an improvement in well-being. Roy herself suggests that one of the main aims of nursing is to promote adaptation in order that the patient may free energy and resources to deal with other stimuli in his or her life. Growth and achievement of well-being may be thought of as maximizing human potential, a process that requires the individual to consume considerable amounts of energy and resources.

Two examples might help. Consider first helping the patient to adapt to giving up smoking; this improves cardiopulmonary function, giving the patient more energy and resources to develop greater levels of fitness and generally feel better. By the same token, helping the patient to adapt successfully to the changes in self-concept involved in stoma formation liberates the patient to resume normal life and develop new roles with confidence. From this standpoint, Roy's model, despite its reactive nature, can be seen as a promising tool for health promotion.

The emphasis of Project 2000 on community care also has implications for curriculum design, since the way nursing is taught must at least in part be applicable to the non-hospital situation. This requires an approach to nursing that recognizes the importance of the patient as at least an equal partner in care and underlines the importance of family and social networks, self-care, independence and successful adaptation to life again after leaving hospital. These of course are the sorts of philosophies that guided King, Orem, Roper and Roy in their models of nursing. This body of ideas is therefore very appropriate to the Project 2000 curriculum.

The nurse tutor using these models must also be aware of the very different care setting that the patient's home may present compared to hospital and be realistic in their use. Atkinson *et al.* (1990) have cautioned against viewing a chaotic set of home circumstances and then saying there is no point in trying to implement a rigid model of nursing to plan care for the unfortunate patient. The patient needs care and care needs planning. In this case a terminally ill young woman with AIDS contracted from IV drug abuse after a chaotic lifestyle involving prostitution and theft to support her drug habit. She was cared for by a large family in the heart of one of Glasgow's most deprived areas and achieved a pain-free death with dignity. The authors point out that they learnt most by listening to the client's and family's needs (staying close to the customer, see p. 9) and by looking for the possibilities for excellence of care rather than the barriers.

The overwhelming view of the literature is that in introducing models a multi-model approach is required (Field, 1987; Botha, 1989; Kristjansen *et al.*, 1987; Hardy, 1986; Hoon, 1986). The nursing curriculum must therefore reflect the full spectrum of models that are in the process of development in order that nurses have the conceptual repertoire they need to deal with the almost unlimited variety of patients and problems that they will encounter in their professional career. To plan a curriculum according to one model only is to invite dogma in through the front door and kick professional freedom out the back. The same comment applies to the delivery of nursing in any health authority or large hospital.

This of course raises the question of who teachers the teachers. Morales-Mann and Logan (1990), in discussing the introduction of a model-based curriculum, have emphasized the need for those teaching models to be fully conversant with them, and highlighted the problems encountered by students who then find themselves in clinical areas which are neither using models nor showing any interest in them. In the United Kingdom this underlines the need for nurse tutors to get to grips with models and how to use them as vehicles for teaching different aspects of nursing.

This latter point is very important because pre-registration students have to learn their nursing skills at the same time as any nursing model. For example, the author teaches surgical nursing using the Roy model to second-year BSc/RGN students. It would be very easy to concentrate on the Roy model at the expense of teaching students how to care for patients undergoing surgery. The balance between the two is crucial; the key is successfully relating the sorts of problems that patients have after (and before) surgery to the Roy approach, demonstrating how Roy's model can help the patient but also being critical of areas where the model might be weak. Nursing models cannot be taught in a vacuum, they must be closely related to areas of clinical nursing.

Nursing education has long been plagued by the difficulties that arise when students find that clinical experience differs substantially from classroom theory. The problems that will arise from teaching models in school that are not practised in the clinical area are therefore nothing new. However, having said that, educationalists cannot walk away from the problem shaking their heads and muttering 'So what's new?'. Whatever model is used, even the traditional medical model, care should benefit from closer links between theory and practice. Joint clinical/educational appointments will help to move education towards practice, but the need remains to move clinical practice towards education.

There is no point teaching anything if the nurse is never going to practise what is taught. This has fundamental implications for Project 2000, for unless nursing practice changes to reflect the new type of practitioner being produced, Project 2000 will be a waste of time, money and nurses as the disillusioned and frustrated nurse leaves the profession. The holistic view of the person, community care, the emphasis on positive health promotion, and nursing models are all included in this statement. Nurses trained under the old system (including the author) need to accept that changes in clinical practice have to happen for a variety of reasons, not least of which is that the professional nurse of the 1990s will be a very different type of nurse from his or her predecessors.

This all leads to the conclusion that changes in nursing practice need changes in education, and changes in education will force changes in practice. One drives the other and closely involved in all these changes will be nursing models. Thus, clinical areas need to invest time and energy in nursing models. Maybe this is unduly optimistic, but without hope why bother getting up in the morning? Changes in practice will have to occur as more and more nurses qualify with a model-based education, hopefully reducing the practice–theory gap that has bedevilled education for so long. The need remains, though, for education to move towards practice at the same time with joint appointments.

In order that a model-based curriculum may be developed, teaching staff need to develop new tools and methods. There needs to be recognition, as Aggleton and Chalmers (1987) point out, that a developmental model requires a different approach to curriculum design from a systems or interactionist model. For example, the developmental approach is concerned with locating blocks to development and other factors that hinder growth and maturation, as well as considering the normal process of ageing from cradle to grave. Social-science teaching needs integrating with the nursing to reflect this approach, while on the other hand anatomy and physiology need teaching with the focus on development (growth and degenerative changes with age) rather than a pure systems approach. Students need to look at their own development in order to better understand that of their patients, which has implications for teaching methods; reflective group work is required rather than formal lectures.

Aggleton and Chalmers have similarly shown the need for systems models to be taught with emphasis on concepts of homeostasis and how systems relate to each other and to nursing care, while the interactionist approach calls for work to identify how individuals feel about their own health, how they construct meaning out of experience, and how they see themselves. This latter approach leans much more heavily on small-group work than the former.

In conclusion, we can see that educationalists need to introduce a variety of models as part of the reform of pre-registration nursing, but should be aware that a lot of careful attention to curriculum design is needed. Integration with practice will be difficult, but is a necessary goal to be striving for since models, and the approach they represent, are a fundamental component of Project 2000. There is no point in practising that which is not taught (traditional medical model) or in teaching that which is not practised (holistic nursing models).

Models and the development of nursing as a profession

Major change and upheaval seem to have become the norm in the delivery of health care in the United Kingdom in the latter part of the 1980s. Government plans make it clear that such radical change is set to continue into the 1990s. Not surprisingly, nursing has been caught up in this veritable whirlwind and must move quickly and positively to adapt to the changing climate we face in the new decade. The question, therefore, must be asked whether the task of developing nursing models will be a help or a hindrance to the nurse, and to the most important group of all, patients.

Gruending (1985) has suggested that the development of nursing models can be seen as a way of professionalizing nursing, although she readily acknowledges that there is little consensus on what exactly constitutes a profession in the first place. On the basis of an analysis of the literature, Gruending offers as a working definition the view that a profession may be seen as a complex, organized occupation whose practitioners have engaged in a lengthy training programme aimed at the acquisition of a specialized body of knowledge. A code of ethics is a key determinant of practice together with regulations enforced by members of the profession which reflect the wishes of the profession. Competence is tested and licensed in the same way.

If this work is set against the views of writers such as Aggleton and Chalmers (1987), who see nursing models as attempts to establish the foundations of a systematic body of knowledge that is uniquely nursing and which has common meaning among nurses, then nursing models are an integral part of the definition of professionalism. The 'specialized body of knowledge' referred to in the preceding paragraph is the stuff of nursing. Nursing models seek to extend knowledge of nursing across nurses, rather than have the situation where each individual practitioner has their own idiosyncratic view of nursing which is not readily accessible to others. For example, saying that Orem's model is probably suitable for planning care for Mrs Smith conveys in a phrase the whole concept of how care should be approached for this patient. However, to describe the Orem model from first principles would take a long time, as long as it might take to describe any other nurse's individual model of care. Nursing models, therefore, are a key ingredient of professionalism in that they give nurses a common set of ideas and concepts that define nursing.

The reader may ask 'Ok, so why be a professional?' The answer is that there are a great many advantages to be conferred on patients by having a profession of nursing, as well as on individual nurses themselves. The presence of a large, responsible and well-trained group of carers in close contact with patients maximizes the quality of health care delivery. It takes more than doctors to have a good health care system!

The recognition of nursing as a profession conveys advantages in terms of prestige, autonomy of practice, public recognition, power and authority. Financial rewards in the United Kingdom have lagged far behind other countries which have a professional nursing service, although the real progress that has been made on salaries in the last few years has been largely due to the skilful harnessing of public recognition and support by organizations such as the Royal College of Nursing and the influence of the Pay Review Body.

The power and autonomy of nursing have been under continual attack since 1985 with the Griffiths Report and the introduction of general management. These changes have systematically removed nursing from the control and management of nurses, leaving the most senior nurse in many areas at ward level. Even the recognized leader of the clinical team, the ward sister/charge nurse, is now being changed by non-nurse senior managers into a ward manager with diminishing clinical responsibility. The next step logically is to remove the requirement for such a person to be a nurse. The old unit system is being replaced by clinical directorates which are usually medically run. The net effect is to strip away the various layers of nursing authority and remove nurses further and further from any position of real power.

Meanwhile, in the community, the GP has been given the lead in care and community nursing services see themselves as being under real threat. The uncertainty has been exacerbated by government attempting to introduce a community care bill against the wishes of the vast majority of the nursing profession. The government then halted the process of change because of the financial consequences and the political repercussions of the substantial increases in the Poll Tax that would have been required to pay for the changes.

The 1990s have therefore opened with nursing under attack. The notion of nurses controlling nursing seems to have been rejected by

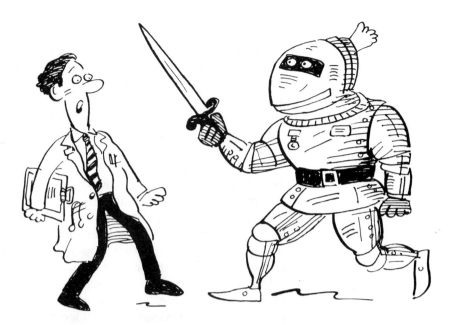

government in favour of nurses doing what they are told by managers and doctors. In effect, one of the fundamental cornerstones of professionalism — autonomy — is being chipped away. Nurses must fight back if they wish to maintain their professional status and do so by establishing the boundaries of nursing expertise and practice.

The views of Gruending (1985) are particularly relevant here, for she has argued that nursing theory works at two levels, the micro and the macro level. Consider an elderly male diabetic patient who, for example, has just returned from theatre after a below-knee amputation. The nurse who carries out a pressure-sore risk assessment using the Norton or Waterlow scale, decides that the patient is at risk, and institutes a 2-hour turning regime with particular attention being paid to pressure relief of areas such as the heels is acting in a logical problem solving and independent way. This nurse is acting at the level of nursing microtheory using nursing knowledge to act independently.

Models act as broad organizing concepts, as philosophies or frameworks of care, and in that sense operate at the large-scale or macro-theory level. In the example above, whether the nurse was using Roy, Orem or any other model to plan care, the problem, goal and interventions would have been largely the same initially. Over a slightly longer timescale Orem's philosophy might have led to more emphasis on encouraging the patient to move himself whereas Roy's approach might have led to using a ripple mattress to help the patient adapt to his immobility. It could be argued, though, that using a ripple mattress also constituted the nurse carrying out the self-care the patient would normally do for himself if able. When considered on the macro scale, models incorporate a substantial amount of nursing microtheory which remains constant from model to model; what

149

differs is the nurse's approach to implementing that theory. In addition, models also take the nurse into broad tracts of territory that do differ with the model, particularly at the assessment stage. For example, Roy leads the nurse to explore self-concept, role function and interdependence but has much less emphasis on the developmental side of the patient that is highlighted by Orem.

In summary, we can say that at the macro level of theory different models place differing emphases on areas of the patient for the nurse to explore. Each model also has its own unique philosophy of care. At the micro level, nursing theory remains an independent body of knowledge, applicable under any model of nursing, but which may be implemented in different ways, subject to the approach of that model. We will return to this issue later as it is of fundamental importance in trying to decide whether models of nursing bring about any improvement in standards of care.

Models, therefore, are essential in defining nursing. Only by saying that 'This is nursing' and that only a trained qualified nurse can do whatever nursing consists of will we be able to hang on to the domain of nursing. Once that is lost an army of low-paid health care assistants (HCAs) acting as 'basic carers' and 'physician's assistants' can be employed to take over. This would be detrimental both to patients and, obviously, to nurses. The huge amount of care provided by informal carers, e.g. family, should not be overlooked in this discussion, and neither should the emphasis placed by some models on the importance of nurses teaching family and others to care for patients. That too becomes part of nursing.

Consider four of the major challenges that face us today, starting with the need for nursing to set standards of care that are measurable in order that patients may receive the quality care they are entitled to. Increasing patient throughput leads to an ever-quickening pace of care delivery to ever more dependent patients. It is likely that this care will be increasingly delivered by health care assistants as students are phased out as part of the workforce with the implementation of Project 2000. Finally, nurses must be able to justify their care to non-nursing management, particularly in terms of cost-effectiveness. These challenges require nursing to respond vigorously.

Nursing models can be a useful part of that response by acting as the cement that holds nursing together. To set a coherent, patient-centred series of standards, requires a philosophy of care, a model of nursing. The rapid throughput of patients and their interaction with a host of professions requires nurses to coordinate what could otherwise become chaos and confusion. It is the nurses who can give the patient a sense of continuity and security. Nursing care must therefore be coherent and consistent, which requires it to be based upon a common approach shared by all nursing staff, i.e. a nursing model implemented with the use of primary nursing.

The employment of large numbers of HCAs could lead to the return of task-oriented care. HCAs will not have the benefit of a nursing education and it is doubtful whether many will have the higher level intellectual skills required for perceptive assessment, deductive thought and the integration of information into planning for and carrying out comprehensive, holistic care. The registered nurse in charge of a 24-bed ward with, say, four HCAs comprising the staff for the shift could be forgiven for feeling that the only way to get the work done was to divide it up into tasks, each HCA doing one or two tasks for everybody, which left the RN free to do the drug round and the difficult dressing on Mr Brown. Would it be fair to expect HCAs to plan integrated care? It certainly would be in breach of the UKCC competencies, which state that is the RN's responsibility. If the HCAs cannot plan integrated care, it is unlikely that they would be able to carry it out with the little supervision that a busy RN could offer in such a situation. If the HCA was able to carry out integrated care, that begs the question of why we should bother with expensive 3-year RN education programmes.

In such a situation we might regress to nursing by the lowest common denominator, i.e. task-oriented care which does not require any integrated view of the person, their health status or the way they interact with the environment and the nurse. These are ideals that we must hang on to if we are to preserve the notion of professional nursing; they are also of course the key components of nursing models.

Cost-cutting management with little knowledge of nursing can cause untold harm. Nursing must stand up to the accountants and performance-related-pay bureaucrats in defence of itself and patients. Clochés like 'We've always done it that way' are no longer any defence. Nursing microtheory and macrotheory must be deployed together, for example, to justify the need for registered nurses to spend time on a busy surgical ward teaching patients pre-operatively. Pre-operative teaching promotes post-operative recovery by reducing anxiety and pain levels (microtheory); this is a desirable goal when an adaptation model of nursing is used (macrotheory). If the nurse can support the microtheory argument with some hard numbers in terms of an estimated reduction in post-operative inpatient days of care required per year and the cost savings involved, she is in a very strong position to argue with any manager who wants to know why the ward needs more than one staff nurse on duty for any shift. The alternative argument, 'We've always had 2 RNs on an early' will not get very far in avoiding the scenario where an HCA is given bed pans, fluids and reassurance as her jobs for the morning.

The issue of professionalism is therefore not about prestige and higher salaries, but rather the survival of nursing itself in an increasingly hostile health care environment. Nurses must be able to show that skilled nursing actually benefits patients. Even then there are further problems to overcome as, sadly, government ideology and political expediency more than ever have come to govern health care in the United Kingdom. Nursing knowledge and nursing models are two of the bastions around which we must build our defence of nursing, for they allow us to define what nursing is. If we lose autonomy, we have lost nursing.

Model testing and development in the 1990s	Keen followers of the very perceptive TV series 'Yes Minister' may feel that the Civil Service is full of people like Sir Humphrey who can always find a great many reasons for never changing anything. The result is a great deal of talk, many papers but little action. The issue of nursing models over the last few years seems to have been treated in the same way in the United Kingdom. A great many people claim to have found reasons why they cannot or should not be implemented, and little actually has been done.

British nursing has been talking for too long about models; it is time to see whether they can be made to work! This book has argued strongly for flexibility, with models being interpreted and developed in the light of practice, while the straitjacket of a one-model-only approach must be avoided. Hanucharurnkul (1989) has given one example of that flexibility in analysing the differences and similarities between Orem and King's models, showing that King stresses nurse–patient interaction and mutual goal setting as distinct from Orem's views, which tend to place the nurse in the dominant role. King is seen as being limited to the areas of patient communication and interrelationships with others while Orem's model has a much broader sweep and strong physiological component.

The two differing stances are, however, eminently compatible and can be brought together, with King's ideas influencing the way the nurse applies Orem's self-care model. Thus, the nurse should be seeking to find out the patients' views of their self-care requisites during the assessment stage and goal setting should be a mutual exercise of equal partners. This hybrid approach might add to Orem's model further themes such as consideration of how well patients can communicate their self-care needs and the effects of patients' environent on their self-care abilities.

As another example of the potential for flexible and creative use of models, the nurse may feel that Roper's concept of independence in activities of daily living is a sound one for the area he or she works in. However, the aspects of the patient that Roper asks the nurse to assess seem to be chosen very arbitrarily, so staff may decide to redesign the assessment tool around a totally different set of headings aiming for a more integrated picture of the patient which describes and analyses psychological and social functioning as well as physical.

The philosophy of care, though, remains that of restoring the maximum amount of independence to the patient. Nurses must be bold and not feel that models are written on tablets of stone; they can be altered and changed according to patient needs.

The Sir Humphreys of the nursing world are quick to point out that nobody has shown that implementing a model of nursing has improved nursing care. This is true, although nobody has shown that a model makes care any worse either! Demonstrating improvements as a result of model implementation is a very difficult task as it involves measuring the quality of nursing care, which still has a large component of subjectivity and is subject to many confounding variables, despite all the work of the past few years on quality control. The problem of a confounding variable is understood as something that might influence the results of a study other than the matter under investigation, in this case a model of nursing. Examples might be differences in patient characteristics or the attitudes and abilities of nursing staff, all of which can affect the outcome of care.

The work of Faucett *et al.* (1990) referred to on p. 31 shows just some of the problems inherent in this work. They discovered that what nurses wrote in their care plans varied little between an experimental ward that was using Orem and a control ward that continued with the institution's traditional methods of nursing. This might mean that the nursing model made no difference to care. There are, however, other interpretations, such as that this merely showed that the institutional habits, conventions and legal requirements were more powerful factors in the writing of care plans than a newly introduced nursing model. Another point of view might be to question the nature of the relationship between what is written and what is done. How closely does a written care plan reflect the care actually given? Might the study have been better observing the nursing care as practised, describing it from a qualitative point of view and then measuring it quantitatively against outcome standards?

Consideration needs to be given to the point of view that perhaps because of the general, philosophical macro level at which nursing models operate, they may not produce change which is readily measurable in patient terms. This is certainly the view of Gruending (1985). There are certainly a great many confounding variables which make such testing a daunting task!

However, at the micro level of nursing theory, empirical testing is possible. The example of the Waterlow pressure-sore risk assessment referred to earlier is a good example; it is an empirically derived tool, and its use can be tested to see whether it improves care by reducing incidence of pressure sores. The reader can think of many examples such as the care of wounds or patient education and teaching which comprise discrete pieces of nursing theory, the value of which can usually be demonstrated. Thus, aspects of nursing theory at micro level can be empirically tested, but perhaps the larger macro scale of nursing models is not amenable to such methods.

This view leads to the conclusion that nursing models are not models in the conventional scientific sense of the word, as then they should be amenable to empirical testing. It seems a paradox that small-scale components of nursing theory can be tested but not the larger-scale ones. But this is not necessarily so: consider the analogy of socialism and capitalism as competing models of political and economic thought. What truly objective data are there to demonstrate that one is beter than the other? If the case was 'provable', perhaps the issue would have been resolved by now, given the passionate arguments of the proponents of these two competing models. If socialism and capitalism represent models of economics on a grand scale (macrotheory), it is also true that on a smaller scale there are elements of economic microtheory that actually are demonstrable and subject to empirical testing and which apply equally well whatever the political ideology of the government; for example, inflation leads to increased wage demands, cutting the price of a product usually increases sales, and raising interest rates usually suppresses demand and cools off an economy.

Perhaps nursing models may best be thought of as subjective views of nursing which by virtue of widespread discussion become generally accepted by nurses, leading to a series of coherent frameworks which have consistent value systems applicable to the delivery of care. There is a nucleus of nursing microtheory applicable under any model of nursing, e.g. 2-hourly turns to relieve pressure, but the way that theory is applied will be influenced and directed by the model of nursing in use. Each model should also lead to the development of its own microtheory. The result is a core of common nursing theory which can be utilized in differing ways according to the model in use, and areas of theory unique to each individual model (see Figure 1).

There are therefore two differing views on the way forward for testing nursing models, one view urging the setting up of trials to try to evaluate their effectiveness and an alternative proposition which states that they are largely untestable in the conventional quantitative way. If the reader adopts the former point of view, it seems that work will have to concentrate on trying to assess care as given and resulting patient benefits (i.e. process and outcome) in carefully controlled studies of the type attempted by Faucett (p. 31).

The alternative point of view begs the question of why we should bother with models at all? How much poorer would economic and political life be without socialist and capitalist alternatives as guiding philosophies, yet who can show empirically that one is better than the other? It is the choice that is crucial, allowing people to decide between alternative ways of running the country they live in. Nursing models provide the same choice, offering alternative but coherent frameworks of care. Model A may be more applicable to some patients than Model B, and better suited to the approach of some nurses than

Figure 1. The rectangle represents all the problems patients may have in their lives. A series of nursing models (macrotheories) are applied to these problems, for simplicity in this diagram only three are used but more could be used. As can be seen, the three nursing models cover various areas of the problem field with a large amount of overlap. The overlap area represents a common core of problems that would be discovered by any of the three models. The goals and interventions for each problem (microtheory) would tend to show differences depending upon the philosophy that drives the model (e.g. self-care or adaptation). There are also areas covered by one model only, indicating that some patient problems would only tend to become explicit with a certain approach to care.

Three models cover a lot more of the problem field than only one,

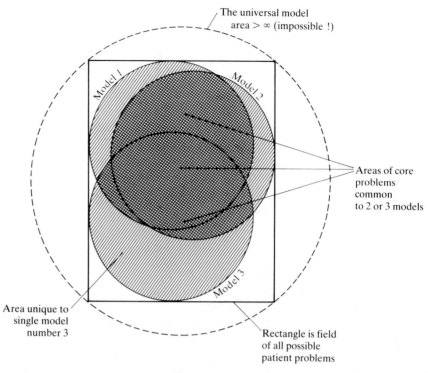

The universal model
area > ∞ (impossible !)

Areas of core
problems
common
to 2 or 3 models

Area unique to
single model
number 3

Rectangle is field
of all possible
patient problems

Each circle is one nursing model

indicating that a series of nursing models are required to deal with the large range of problems a person faces as they pass through their life. It can be seen, therefore, that this approach is preferable to the single-model approach that would leave large areas uncovered.

A universal nursing model would have to encompass the entire rectangle as shown by the dotted circle. However, as the field of possible problems is infinitely large, so the circle drawn around it would have to have an area larger than infinity,

which is impossible by definition, as nothing can be larger than infinity. Whether the nurse uses a common-sense definition, or engages in a little geometry, the result is the same, a universal model of nursing is impossible!

others. What matters is that the choice is there, for both patients and nurses, of different approaches to care. The fact that these approaches provide a common language of concepts and ideas across nurses, can be used for curriculum construction, and may generate new thought and research into nursing is a bonus.

However, neither patients nor nurses will reap any of these potential benefits if nurses do not attempt to use models. They will be of little value if they remain only in the pages of textbooks such as this and others. The time has come for nurses to grasp the nettle of nursing models, to stop talking and finding excuses to do nothing; the time has come for serious attempts at making them work in practice as organizing tools for the developing body of nursing microtheory. The alternative is that nursing will lose its autonomy, being relegated to the grade of physician's assistant. If nurses want a job description that consists of doing all the bits and pieces nobody else wants to do, then many nurses need to recognize that current practice and attitudes are leading in that direction. Only by saying 'This is nursing!' and fighting for what we believe in can we defend ourselves and patients from the deskilling and fragmentation of care that current trends are producing. The implementation and development of nursing models could provide nurses with powerful ammunition for the conflicts that lie ahead. Few battles are won with an empty arsenal.

References

Aggleton P & Chalmers H (1987) Models of nursing, nursing practice and nurse educations. *Journal of Advanced Nursing,* **12**, 573–581.

Atkinson J, Mackay E & Robertson G (1990) Own home, own bed, own life. *Nursing Standard,* **4**(4), 48–49.

Botha E (1989) Theory development in perspective; the role of conceptual frameworks and models in theory development. *Journal of Advanced Nursing,* **14**, 49–55.

Brubaker B (1983) Health promotion: a linguistic analysis. *Advances in Nursing Science,* **5**(3), 1–14.

Dunn B (1990) Health promotion and Orem's model. *Nursing Standard,* **4**(40), 34.

Faucett J, Ellis V, Underwood P, Naqvi A & Wilson D (1990) The effect of Orem's self care model on nursing care in a nursing home setting. *Journal of Advanced Nursing,* **15**, 659–666.

Field PA (1987) The impact of nursing theory on clinical decision making process. *Journal of Advanced Nursing,* **12**, 563–571.

Gruending DL (1985) Nursing theory: a vehicle of professionalisation. *Journal of Advanced Nursing,* **10**, 553–558.

Hardy L (1986) Identifying the place of theoretical frameworks in an evolving discipline. *Journal of Advanced Nursing,* **11**, 103–107.

Hartweg D (1990) Health promotion self care within Orem's general theory of nursing. *Journal of Advanced Nursing,* **15**, 35–41.

Hanucharurnkul S (1989) Comparative analysis of Orem's and King's theories. *Journal of Advanced Nursing,* **14**, 365–372.

Hoon E (1986) Game playing; a way to look at nursing models. *Journal of Advanced Nursing,* **11**, 421–427.

Kristjansen L, Tamblyn R & Kuypers J (1987) A model to guide development and application of multiple nursing theories. *Journal of Advanced Nursing,* **12**, 523–529.

Morales-Mann ETG & Logan M (1990) Implementing the Roy model; challenges for nurse educators. *Journal of Advanced Nursing,* **15**, 142–147.

Pender NJ (1984) Health promotion and illness prevention. In Wevley H & Fitzpatrick J (eds) *Annual Review of Nursing Research,* vol. 2, pp. 83–105. New York: Springer.

Pender NJ (1987) *Health Promoition in Nursing Practice.* Norwalk, Conn.: Appleton and Lange.

Rambo BJ (1984) *Adaptation Nursing: Assessment and Intervention.* Philadelphia: W.B. Saunders.

Index

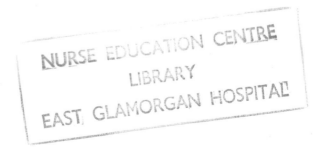